Somatic Exercises for Beginners

Transform Your Life in 30 Days with Personalized Exercises for Body and Mind

Owen Mark Artisan

ISBN-- 9781738553327

Disclaimer: The information provided in the book "Somatic Exercises for Beginners: Transform Your Life in 30 Days with Personalized Exercises for Body and Mind" is intended for educational and informational purposes only. The exercises and guidance offered are not a substitute for professional medical advice, diagnosis, or treatment. Readers are advised to consult with their healthcare provider or a qualified professional before beginning any new exercise program or making significant lifestyle changes. The author and publisher of this book are not liable for any injuries, damages, or consequences resulting from the use of the exercises or information presented within. Individual results may vary, and it is recommended to approach the exercises with caution, taking into consideration one's own physical and mental well-being.

The names mentioned in this content are entirely fictional and have been crafted solely for the purpose of creative expression and narrative context. These names are not intended to depict, imitate, or reference any real individuals, organizations, events, or locations. Any similarities to actual entities are purely coincidental

Contents

Introduction

Welcome to Somatic Wellness

Hello there, and a warm welcome to your journey towards a happier, healthier you! If you've picked up this book, chances are you're on a quest to find balance and harmony within your body and mind. You're in just the right place. Imagine we're sitting down together, sipping on our favorite beverages, embarking on a conversation that could very well transform the way you live your life. That's the spirit of this journey we're about to take together.

Somatic wellness might sound like a complex term, but at its heart, it's beautifully simple. It's about reconnecting with your body, listening to its whispers (and sometimes, its loud demands), and learning how to move and rest in ways that nourish your entire being. It's the art of tuning in to the subtle signals your body sends you, signals that, in our busy lives, we often overlook or silence.

Think of your body as a wise friend who's been with you through every high and low, always ready to offer support. But, like in any friendship, communication is key. Somatic wellness teaches us to engage in a deep and meaningful dialogue with our bodies. Through gentle, personalized exercises that blend physical movements with mindfulness, we learn to understand and care for our bodies, leading to profound changes not just physically, but emotionally and mentally as well.

This book is your guide to a 30-day transformation, a journey designed to introduce you to the principles of somatic wellness and to help you craft a personalized plan that fits your unique needs. Whether you're dealing with stress, looking to alleviate pain, or simply wishing to enhance your overall wellbeing, you'll find tools and practices here that will speak directly to you.

And the best part? You don't need to be an expert in anything to start. All you need is a willingness to listen, to explore, and to gently experiment with the practices shared in these pages. Together, we'll discover how small, mindful changes can lead to big transformations, not just for the next 30 days, but for life.

So, let's begin this journey with an open heart and an open mind, ready to embrace the changes and challenges that lie ahead. Remember, this is not just about the destination but about the beautiful discoveries we'll make along the way. Welcome to the world of somatic wellness. I'm so glad you're here.

Understanding Somatic Exercises

Imagine your body is like a garden. Just as a garden needs regular tending—watering, weeding, and sunlight—to thrive, your body needs care and attention to flourish. Somatic exercises are the gardening tools in your wellness toolkit, designed to nurture and maintain your body's well-being.

So, what exactly are somatic exercises? In simple terms, they're movements and practices that focus on the internal experience of moving—how it feels rather than how it looks. It's not about lifting the heaviest weights at the gym or running the fastest mile. Instead, it's about moving with awareness and intention, tuning in to the sensations in your body, and fostering a deeper connection between your mind and body.

Think of somatic exercises as learning to dance by listening to the music inside you rather than following strict steps. It's about moving in a way that feels good and right for you, exploring and adjusting as you go. These exercises teach you to listen to your body's signals—a tightness here, a discomfort there—and respond with movements that release tension and restore balance.

For example, if you've ever stretched in the morning, reaching your arms wide or arching your back, and felt a sense of relief and readiness for the day, you've touched on the essence of somatic exercises. It's about finding those natural, intuitive movements that help your body feel its best.

In our journey through somatic wellness, we'll explore various exercises that help you reconnect with your body's natural rhythms and wisdom. Whether it's through gentle stretching, conscious breathing, or mindful movement, you'll learn to cultivate a sense of ease and well-being that permeates your entire life.

Just as a gardener learns to understand the needs of each plant, through somatic exercises, you'll learn to understand and attend to the needs of your body. And just like a well-tended garden blooms beautifully, a body nurtured through somatic practices blossoms into its fullest potential of health and happiness.

Let's dive a bit deeper into the essence of somatic exercises by expanding on this garden analogy. Imagine each part of your body as a different plant in your garden. Some plants might need more sunlight, while others thrive in the shade. Similarly, different parts of your body have unique needs for movement and rest. Somatic exercises help you tune into these needs, allowing you to provide the right kind of care—just like deciding when to water your plants or when to let them soak up the sun.

One key aspect of somatic exercises is mindfulness—being fully present in the moment. Imagine you're watering your garden. Instead of doing it absentmindedly, you pay attention to each plant, noticing its leaves, its growth, and how the water absorbs into the soil. Similarly, with somatic exercises, you're fully present with each movement, noticing how your muscles stretch, how your breath flows, and how your body feels with each motion. This mindfulness creates a deep connection between your mind and body, leading to a harmonious inner garden.

Somatic exercises also emphasize the quality of movement over quantity. It's not about doing a hundred repetitions mindlessly but about performing a few movements with full awareness and attention. Think of pruning a bush in your garden. It's not about how many branches you cut but about which branches you choose to prune to allow the plant to grow more healthily. In the same way, somatic exercises focus on the quality of each movement to ensure that your body benefits fully from each practice.

Adaptability is another cornerstone of somatic exercises. Just as a garden changes with the seasons, your body's needs can change from day to day. What felt good yesterday might not feel the same today, and that's okay. Somatic exercises teach you to listen to your body and adapt your movements accordingly, just like adjusting your gardening techniques to the changing seasons.

Lastly, the goal of somatic exercises is to cultivate a sense of well-being that permeates your entire life, much like a well-tended garden brings beauty and joy not just to the gardener but to everyone who sees it. By learning to listen to and care for your body through these exercises, you're not just improving your physical health but also enhancing your emotional and mental well-being. It's about creating a vibrant inner landscape that supports you in living your life with more joy, ease, and fulfillment.

In summary, somatic exercises are your tools for nurturing the garden of your body. They encourage mindfulness, quality of movement, adaptability, and an overall sense of well-being. As you embark on this journey, remember that you are both the gardener and the garden, and through somatic practices, you have the power to cultivate a thriving, beautiful space within yourself.

The 30-Day Transformation

Embarking on a 30-day journey to transform your life might sound like a tall order, but imagine it as a gentle path through a serene and beautiful landscape, rather than a steep climb up a mountain. This book is designed to guide you through each step of that path, making the journey not only manageable but also deeply rewarding. Let's break down how we'll navigate this journey together, ensuring you feel supported and motivated every step of the way.

Week 1: Awakening the Body

In the first week, think of yourself as a gardener taking stock of their garden after a long winter. We'll start by gently awakening your body, introducing somatic exercises that help you tune in to your physical sensations and begin to nurture your body-mind connection. Each day, you'll explore simple movements and mindfulness practices that open the door to somatic awareness, laying the groundwork for the transformative journey ahead.

Week 2: Building Strength and Flexibility

As your awareness deepens, we'll start to cultivate your inner garden, focusing on building strength and flexibility. This week is about planting seeds that will grow into robust plants. Through a carefully selected series of exercises, you'll start to build the physical and mental resilience needed for a flourishing life. These practices are designed to be accessible, allowing you to progress at your own pace and adapt exercises to suit your body's needs.

Week 3: Enhancing Emotional Balance

By the third week, you'll be tending to the blossoming flowers of your garden—your emotions. This week introduces somatic practices that help you connect with your emotional landscape, offering tools for managing stress, anxiety, and other emotional challenges. Like learning to balance the ecosystem of a garden, you'll explore how to cultivate emotional balance, fostering a sense of calm and resilience that supports your overall well-being.

Week 4: Integrating Somatic Wellness into Daily Life

In the final week, you'll learn to sustain your blooming garden, integrating somatic wellness into your daily life. This week is about turning the practices and insights gained over the past 30 days into sustainable habits. You'll discover advanced techniques for maintaining your somatic wellness and adapting your personal practice to continue supporting your journey beyond this month.

Conclusion: Reflecting and Continuing Your Journey

As we reach the end of our 30-day transformation, we'll take time to reflect on the journey and celebrate your growth. You'll be invited to envision the future of your inner garden and how you can continue nurturing it. The conclusion offers encouragement and guidance for maintaining your somatic wellness practice as an ongoing journey of self-discovery and growth.

Throughout this book, each day offers a step-by-step guide, complete with exercises, reflections, and tips for integrating somatic wellness into your life. You're encouraged to approach this journey with curiosity, openness, and compassion for yourself. Remember, transformation is not about achieving perfection; it's about growth, learning, and finding joy in the process.

Welcome to your 30-day transformation. Your path to somatic wellness starts here, and I'm thrilled to be guiding you through this rewarding journey. Together, we'll discover the power of listening to your body, embracing change, and cultivating a life of wellness and harmony. Let's begin.

Part I: Foundations of Somatic Wellness

Chapter 1: The Somatic Mind-Body Connection

The science behind somatic practices.

The science behind somatic practices illuminates the profound impact these methods have on our health and well-being, bridging the gap betwèen our physical sensations and mental states. Somatic practices, encompassing a range of activities from yoga and meditation to mindful movement and breathwork, tap into the body's inherent ability to heal and restore itself. Let's explore the key scientific principles that underpin these transformative practices.

1. The Autonomic Nervous System and Homeostasis

The autonomic nervous system (ANS) plays a critical role in regulating our body's unconscious actions, such as heart rate, digestion, and respiratory rate. Somatic practices influence the ANS, particularly its two main branches: the sympathetic nervous system (SNS), which governs the body's stress response ('fight or flight'), and the parasympathetic nervous system (PNS), which controls the body's rest and digest functions.

Engaging in somatic exercises can shift the balance from the SNS to the PNS, promoting relaxation and reducing stress. For example, deep breathing exercises slow the heart rate and lower blood pressure, signaling the body to enter a state of calm. This shift helps restore homeostasis, or balance, within the body, enhancing overall health and resilience.

2. The Mind-Body Connection

The concept of the mind-body connection is central to understanding how somatic practices work. This connection is mediated through various physiological pathways, including the endocrine (hormonal) system and the immune system. Stressful thoughts and emotions can trigger the release of stress hormones like cortisol, which have physical effects on the body. Conversely, physical movements and relaxation techniques can produce psychological benefits by reducing levels of stress hormones and increasing the production of mood-enhancing neurotransmitters like serotonin and dopamine.

Research in psychoneuroimmunology (PNI) further explores how the brain, nervous system, and immune system interact, showing that mental states can influence immune function. Somatic practices, by improving mental well-being, can therefore enhance immune response and reduce the risk of illness.

3. Neuroplasticity and Somatic Experiences

Neuroplasticity refers to the brain's ability to form and reorganize synaptic connections, especially in response to learning or experience. Somatic practices leverage this principle by creating new, positive body-mind connections. Through repeated, mindful engagement in somatic exercises, individuals can rewire their brains to respond differently to stress, pain, and emotional challenges.

For instance, mindfulness meditation has been shown to increase the density of gray matter in parts of the brain associated with attention, emotional regulation, and self-awareness. Similarly, movement-based practices like yoga can alter brain structures that control stress and anxiety, offering lasting benefits to mental health.

4. The Role of the Vagus Nerve

The vagus nerve is a key component of the PNS and plays a pivotal role in the body's relaxation responses. It extends from the brainstem to the abdomen, innervating various organs along the way. Somatic practices that involve deep breathing, gentle stretching, and relaxation techniques can activate the vagus nerve, promoting a state of calm and reducing stress and inflammation throughout the body.

Stimulation of the vagus nerve also enhances vagal tone, a measure of the body's ability to efficiently return to a state of rest after stress. High vagal tone is associated with better emotional regulation, lower levels of inflammation, and improved resilience to stress.

In Summary

The science behind somatic practices reveals a complex interplay between the body, mind, and nervous system. By engaging in these practices, individuals can tap into their body's natural mechanisms for stress relief, emotional regulation, and self-healing. This scientific understanding not only validates the efficacy of somatic practices but also encourages a holistic approach to health, emphasizing the integration of body and mind in the pursuit of wellness.

Body, Mind, and Emotional health

Welcome to the heart of your journey towards somatic wellness. Imagine your body and mind as lifelong dance partners, constantly in communication, affecting each other's moves. This chapter is all about exploring that intricate dance, using stories and examples that shine a light on how deeply interconnected our physical selves and our mental states truly are.

The Dance of Stress and Relaxation

Let's start with a story about Alex. Alex, a graphic designer, often found themselves overwhelmed with deadlines. Sitting for hours in front of the computer, shoulders tensed, breath shallow, the stress wasn't just in their mind; it was manifesting in their body. One evening, Alex attended a somatic yoga class. Through gentle movements and focused breathing, they noticed something remarkable: as their body relaxed, so did their mind. This wasn't magic; it was the mind-body connection in action. Alex's story beautifully illustrates how stress isn't just a mental experience; it tightens our muscles, quickens our breath, and can even change our posture.

The Power of a Deep Breath

Have you ever noticed how a deep breath can feel like a mini-vacation for your brain? There's a reason for that. Consider Maria, a school teacher, who used deep breathing as a tool to manage classroom chaos. Whenever the noise level rose, instead of raising her voice, she'd take a deep, intentional breath. This simple act didn't just calm her; it set a tone for the whole class. Maria's deep breath was a signal, a physical way to bring peace to a hectic environment. This example shows us how our physical responses can directly influence our emotional state and even affect those around us.

The Feedback Loop

Think of your mind and body as participants in a continuous feedback loop. When Neil, a retired veteran, began experiencing nightmares, his sleep suffered. This lack of rest wasn't just making him tired; it was making his body ache. With the help of a therapist, Neil started practicing mindfulness meditation. As his mind learned to find calm, his sleep improved, and so did his physical pain. Neil's journey underscores the feedback loop between our mental and physical health; improvement in one area can lead to positive changes in the other.

Embodying Confidence

Ever heard the advice to "stand tall" before a big presentation? There's wisdom in that suggestion. Sophia, an aspiring novelist, felt a wave of insecurity before her first public reading. A friend suggested she practice power poses beforehand, standing in a posture of confidence for a few minutes. Sophia was skeptical, but she tried it. To her surprise, not only did she feel more confident, but her audience responded to her with more enthusiasm. Sophia's experience is a testament to how our body language can influence our mental state, affecting how we feel and how others perceive us.

The Healing Walk of Thomas

Thomas, a corporate lawyer, found himself enveloped in stress and anxiety, a common scenario in his high-stakes profession. His weekends were spent ruminating over cases, leading to tension headaches and chronic back pain. One afternoon, heeding the advice of a friend, Thomas took a long walk in the nearby park, focusing on the rhythm of his steps and the beauty around him. Surprisingly, he returned not just with a clearer mind but noticed a significant reduction in his physical discomfort. Thomas's story highlights how physical activity, like walking, can serve as a therapeutic bridge, easing mental stress and consequently alleviating physical ailments.

Jenna's Dance of Liberation

Jenna, a stay-at-home mom, struggled with feelings of isolation and depression. With little time for herself, her emotional state began to manifest physically as lethargy and a constant sense of fatigue. On a whim, she joined a local dance class, a childhood passion long forgotten. The act of dancing, moving her body to the music, and expressing herself without words reignited a spark within her. Jenna's mood lifted, and her energy levels soared. This transformation underscores the power of physical expression in unlocking emotional freedom and vitality.

The Recovery of Ethan

Ethan, an avid runner, faced a major setback when he sustained a knee injury, halting his ability to engage in the activity that was his main stress reliever. The injury not only affected him physically but plunged him into a state of mild depression. During his recovery, Ethan discovered swimming as an alternative. The rhythmic nature of swimming and the sensation of being supported by water helped him find a new form of meditation and relaxation. Ethan's story is a testament to the adaptability of the mind-body connection and the importance of finding alternative pathways to maintain this balance in the face of challenges.

Lily's Garden of Serenity

Lily, a retired school principal, experienced the onset of anxiety as she transitioned into retirement, a common phase where the sudden lack of routine can feel unsettling. Her anxiety manifested physically as insomnia and digestive issues. On her daughter's suggestion, Lily took up gardening, a hobby she had always been curious about but never had the time to explore. The tactile experience of soil, the focus required to plant and nurture, and the satisfaction of watching her garden grow became a therapeutic routine for Lily. Her physical symptoms began to ease as she found peace and a new sense of purpose in her garden. Lily's story illustrates how engaging with nature and physical hobbies can harmonize our internal states, promoting both physical and mental well-being.

In Summary

The stories of Alex, Maria, Neil,Sophia, Thomas, Jenna, Ethan, and Lily serve as windows into the somatic mind-body connection. They teach us that our thoughts, emotions, and physical sensations are not isolated; they're deeply intertwined. This chapter lays the foundation for understanding how, by tuning into this connection, we can harness the power of somatic exercises to transform not just our bodies, but our minds and emotional well-being too.

As we move forward, remember these stories. They're not just tales; they're reflections of the profound impact somatic practices can have on our lives. By embracing this mind-body connection, you're taking the first step toward a holistic approach to wellness, where every movement, every breath, and every moment of mindfulness brings you closer to a state of harmony and health.

Chapter 2: Assessing Your Wellness Needs

Assessing Your Wellness Needs

Welcome to a pivotal step in your journey toward somatic wellness: understanding and assessing your unique wellness needs. This chapter is designed to guide you through a simple, yet profound, self-assessment process. By the end, you'll have a clearer picture of where you are now and where you'd like to be in terms of your physical, emotional, and mental health. Let's embark on this exploration with kindness towards ourselves, remembering that self-awareness is the first step toward transformation.

Step 1: Setting the Stage for Self-Reflection

Before diving into the assessment, find a quiet, comfortable space where you can reflect without interruptions. You might want to have a journal or notebook handy to jot down your thoughts and observations. Approach this process with an open heart and a non-judgmental mind. Remember, this isn't about critiquing yourself; it's about understanding yourself.

Step 2: Reflecting on Your Physical Health

- **Physical Activity**: Think about your current level of physical activity. How often do you move your body in a way that feels good? This isn't just about exercise; consider all forms of movement, from walking to gardening to dancing in your living room.

- **Body Awareness**: Consider how connected you feel to your body. Do you notice when you're tense, relaxed, energized, or tired? How well do you understand your body's signals?

- **Physical Discomfort or Pain**: Reflect on any physical discomfort or pain you experience. Where in your body do you feel it? When does it occur, and what do you think might be contributing factors?

Step 3: Exploring Your Emotional Well-being

- **Stress Levels**: Assess your current stress levels. What are the sources of stress in your life? How do you usually cope with stress?

- **Emotional Awareness**: How in touch are you with your emotions? Can you easily identify what you're feeling and why? How comfortable are you with expressing your emotions?

- **Joy and Fulfillment**: Think about what brings you joy and fulfillment. Are these elements present in your daily life? How often do you engage in activities that make you feel alive and content?

Step 4: Considering Your Mental Health

- **Mindfulness and Presence**: Reflect on your ability to stay present. How often do you find your mind wandering to the past or the future? Do you feel like you're living in the moment?

- **Mental Clutter**: Consider the amount of mental clutter you carry. This can include worries, unresolved issues, or anything that takes up mental space and energy.

- **Self-Care Practices**: Evaluate your current self-care practices. How do you take care of your mental and emotional health? What practices help you feel balanced and centered?

Step 5: Creating Your Wellness Vision

Now that you've reflected on your physical, emotional, and mental health, it's time to envision your ideal state of wellness. Imagine a version of yourself who is thriving in all these areas. What does that look like? How do you feel in this envisioned state? Write down your wellness vision, focusing on the positive changes you wish to see.

Step 6: Setting Intentions

Based on your self-assessment and wellness vision, set a few intentions for your somatic wellness journey. These aren't strict goals but gentle directions you'd like to move towards. Perhaps you want to develop a deeper connection with your body, manage stress more effectively, or cultivate joy and fulfillment. Write these intentions down, framing them in a positive, affirming way.

Step 7: Identifying Your Support System

As you continue your journey toward somatic wellness, it's important to consider the role of support in your life. Reflect on the following:

- **Community and Relationships**: Who in your life supports your wellness journey? This could be friends, family, a support group, or even a health professional.

- **Resources**: What resources do you have access to that can support your journey? Think about books, online communities, local classes, or apps that align with your wellness vision.

- **Asking for Help**: How comfortable are you with asking for help or support? Recognize that reaching out is a strength, not a weakness.

Step 8: Evaluating Your Environment

Your environment plays a crucial role in your wellness. Assess your physical and social environments by considering:

- **Physical Space**: Does your living space support your wellness goals? Think about the presence of nature, the setup of your relaxation or workout area, and the overall vibe of your home.

- **Social Environment**: Assess the impact of your social interactions on your wellness. Are they uplifting and supportive, or do they often leave you feeling drained?

Step 9: Acknowledging Your Achievements

As you reflect on your wellness needs, it's also vital to acknowledge the steps you've already taken towards improving your well-being. Consider:

- **Past Efforts**: Reflect on what you've tried in the past. What worked well for you? What did you enjoy?
- **Learning from Experiences**: What have these efforts taught you about what you need and what you respond to positively?

Step 10: Committing to Exploration and Openness

The final step in assessing your wellness needs is committing to an attitude of exploration and openness as you embark on this journey:

- **Willingness to Try**: Encourage yourself to be open to trying new somatic practices, even if they're outside your comfort zone.
- **Adaptability**: Recognize that your needs and preferences may evolve, and be willing to adapt your approach accordingly.

- **Curiosity**: Approach this journey with curiosity rather than judgment, viewing each experience as an opportunity to learn more about yourself.

Bringing It All Together

Having gone through these steps, you've laid a solid foundation for your somatic wellness journey. You've gained insights into your physical, emotional, and mental health needs, considered your environment and support system, and set intentions that will guide your path forward. Remember, this assessment is not a one-time task but a continuous process of self-discovery and growth.

As you move into the next chapters and start incorporating personalized somatic exercises into your life, keep referring back to your assessments and intentions. They will serve as your compass, helping you navigate your journey with purpose and clarity. Embrace this process with kindness, patience, and a spirit of adventure. Your journey toward somatic wellness is uniquely yours, and every step forward is a step toward a more balanced, healthy, and fulfilled self.

Next Steps

Armed with a deeper understanding of your wellness needs and a clear vision for your journey, you're now ready to delve into the heart of somatic practices. The following chapters will introduce you to a variety of exercises and techniques, each designed to nurture your mind-body connection and support your wellness goals. Remember, this journey is about progress, not perfection. Celebrate each step, stay curious, and let your personal path to somatic wellness unfold.

In Closing

Congratulations on completing your wellness needs assessment! This process of self-reflection is a powerful step toward understanding yourself better and setting the stage for meaningful change. Remember, somatic wellness is a personal journey, and you've just mapped out your starting point. With this foundation, you're ready to explore personalized exercises and practices that resonate with your unique needs and aspirations. Keep your assessments, wellness vision, and intentions close as they will guide you through the transformative days ahead.

Customizing Your 30-Day Somatic Wellness Plan

Creating a personalized 30-day somatic wellness plan is an empowering step toward realizing your health and wellness goals. This plan will be your roadmap, guiding you through exercises and practices tailored to your unique needs, as identified in your self-assessment. Let's embark on this journey with optimism, remembering that every small step contributes to significant transformation.

Step 1: Review Your Assessment Outcomes

Begin by reviewing the insights from your wellness needs assessment. Identify key areas you'd like to focus on, such as reducing stress, enhancing physical flexibility, improving emotional well-being, or fostering mindfulness. These areas will be the cornerstone of your plan.

Step 2: Set Clear, Achievable Goals

For each area you've chosen to focus on, set specific, achievable goals. If you're aiming to reduce stress, a goal might be to practice deep breathing exercises for 10 minutes daily. Ensure your goals are realistic and measurable, so you can track your progress.

Step 3: Choose Your Somatic Practices

Based on your goals, select somatic exercises and practices that align with your needs. Consider a mix of physical activities (like yoga, tai chi, or gentle stretching), mindfulness practices (such as meditation or guided imagery), and emotional wellness techniques (like journaling or emotional freedom technique). Aim for variety to keep your plan engaging and comprehensive.

Step 4: Structure Your Daily Routine

Divide your goals into daily actions. A well-balanced day might include a morning mindfulness practice, midday stretches, and an evening gratitude journal entry. Schedule your activities at times when you're most likely to follow through. Remember, consistency is key, but flexibility is also important. Listen to your body and mind, and adjust as needed.

Step 5: Prepare Your Space and Tools

Create a dedicated space for your somatic practices. It doesn't have to be large—a corner of a room or a quiet spot will do. Gather any tools you might need, such as a yoga mat, meditation cushion, or journal. Having a physical space and the right tools can enhance your commitment and experience.

Step 6: Implement, Reflect, and Adjust

Start implementing your plan, focusing on one day at a time. At the end of each day or week, reflect on what worked well and what didn't. This reflection will help you adjust your plan to better suit your needs. Maybe you find morning yoga invigorating or prefer journaling at night. Tailor your activities to what feels most beneficial.

Step 7: Celebrate Progress

Celebrate your milestones and progress, no matter how small. Acknowledging your efforts reinforces positive behavior and keeps you motivated. Whether it's completing a week of mindfulness practice or noticing a decrease in stress levels, every achievement is worth celebrating.

Step 8: Stay Flexible and Open

Your needs may change as you progress through your 30-day plan, and that's perfectly okay. Stay open to modifying your plan, experimenting with new practices, or adjusting your goals. The aim is to find what best supports your wellness journey, not to stick rigidly to a predetermined path.

Step 9: Integrate Mindfulness into Daily Activities

Beyond scheduled practices, look for opportunities to incorporate mindfulness into your routine activities. Whether it's mindful eating, taking a mindful walk, or practicing deep breathing during work breaks, these moments can significantly enhance your overall sense of well-being.

- **Action Tip**: Choose one routine activity each week to do mindfully. Notice the textures, sounds, and sensations involved, fully engaging with the present moment.

Step 10: Connect with Nature

Nature has a profound effect on somatic wellness, reducing stress and improving mood. Incorporate outdoor activities into your plan, such as walking, gardening, or simply sitting in a park.

- **Action Tip**: Schedule regular time outdoors, even if it's just a few minutes a day, to connect with the natural world and ground yourself.

Step 11: Explore Somatic Movement

Somatic movement focuses on internal perception and experience. Explore practices like Feldenkrais, Alexander Technique, or gentle dance movements to deepen your body awareness and enhance physical and emotional integration.

- **Action Tip**: Dedicate one session each week to exploring a somatic movement practice, focusing on how it feels rather than how it looks.

Step 12: Engage in Social Wellness

Wellness is also about our connections with others. Engage in activities that foster positive interactions, such as joining a wellness group, attending workshops, or practicing somatic exercises with a friend.

- **Action Tip**: Identify one social wellness activity you can participate in each week. It could be as simple as sharing your wellness journey with a friend or joining an online community.

Step 13: Listen and Adapt

As you progress, stay attuned to your body's and mind's responses to different practices. Your plan should be flexible, adapting to what you learn about yourself through this process.

- **Action Tip**: Keep a weekly log of your experiences, noting what feels nourishing and what doesn't. Use this feedback to adjust your plan moving forward.

Step 14: Incorporate Rest and Reflection

Rest is an essential part of somatic wellness. Ensure your plan includes adequate rest, along with time for reflection, to integrate your experiences and insights.

- **Action Tip**: Schedule brief daily periods of rest or reflection. Use this time to meditate, journal, or simply be in silence, allowing your experiences to assimilate.

Step 15: Extend Your Vision Beyond 30 Days

While this plan focuses on the next 30 days, consider how you can sustain and build upon these practices long-term. Wellness is a lifelong journey, not a destination.

- **Action Tip**: At the end of your 30 days, set aside time to reflect on your journey and plan forward. What practices do you want to continue? What new areas of wellness are you curious about?

Bringing It All Together

Your customized 30-day somatic wellness plan is a living document, one that supports and adapts to your journey toward holistic health. Remember, the goal is not perfection but growth and self-discovery. Approach each day with curiosity and kindness, allowing your experiences to guide your path forward. You're not just following a plan; you're nurturing a deeper connection with yourself, cultivating a practice that can support you well beyond these 30 days. Welcome to your journey of transformation.

Final Thoughts

Your 30-day somatic wellness plan is just the beginning. It's a launchpad for a deeper exploration of the interconnectedness of your body, mind, and spirit. By engaging with this plan actively and reflectively, you're not only enhancing your present well-being but also laying the groundwork for sustained health and happiness. Remember, the most powerful aspect of somatic wellness is its capacity to evolve with you, offering endless opportunities for discovery and growth. Embrace this journey with an open heart and mind, and let your experiences guide you toward a deeper understanding and appreciation of your unique path to wellness.

Part II: The Somatic Wellness Program

Chapter 3: Week 1 - Awakening the Body

Welcome to Week 1

Hello there! Welcome to the first week of your somatic wellness journey. Think of me as your guide, walking beside you as we embark on this path together. This week, we're focusing on awakening your body, tuning into its subtle signals, and beginning to move in ways that feel nourishing and revitalizing. Let's dive in with curiosity and an open heart.

Day 1: Grounding and Centering

- **Morning Ritual (Duration: 5 minutes)**: Find a quiet spot where you won't be disturbed. Stand or sit in a comfortable position, plant your feet firmly on the ground, and close your eyes. Take three deep, intentional breaths. As you inhale and exhale, visualize roots extending from the soles of your feet into the earth, anchoring you. Feel the sense of stability and presence this brings.

Tip: If standing is uncomfortable, sitting works just as well. The key is to feel supported and connected to the ground beneath you.

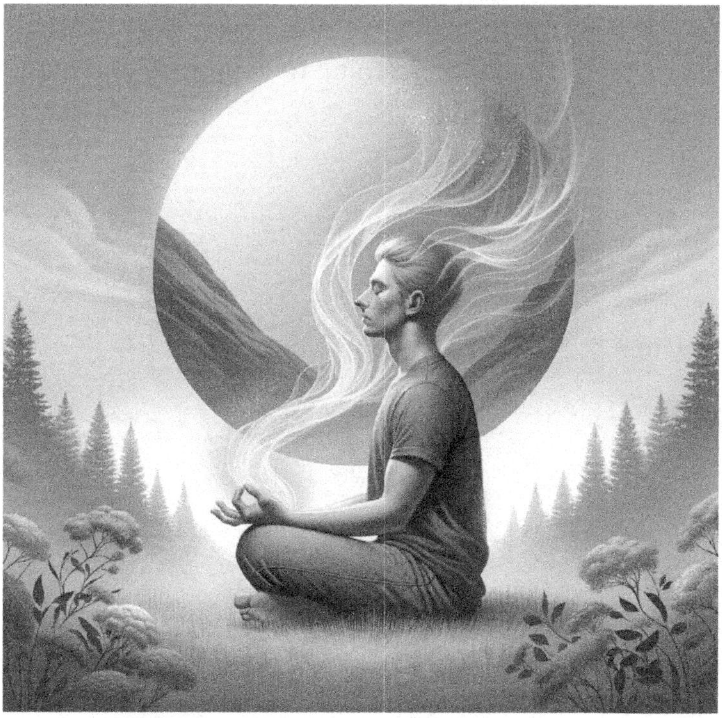

Here's the image illustrating a serene and calming scene, capturing the essence of tranquility and mindfulness

Day 2: Exploring Gentle Movement

- **Midday Break (Duration: 10 minutes)**: Take a moment to stand up from your work or sitting area. Begin with shoulder rolls, slowly bringing awareness to any areas of tension. Proceed with gentle neck stretches, tilting your head from side to side. Finally, let your arms float up above your head and sway gently side to side, imagining you're underwater and your arms are seaweed.

Adjustment: Feel free to adjust the movements to what feels right. This is about listening to your body and moving in a way that feels good.

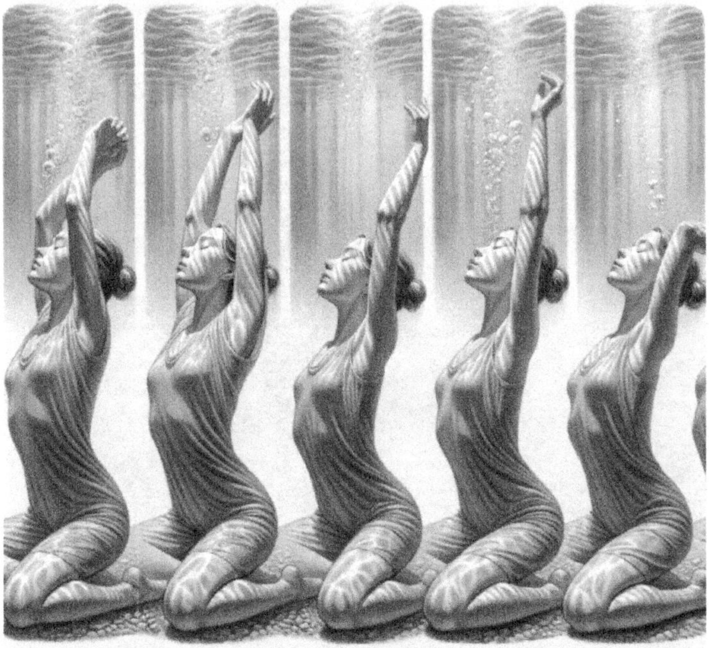

The image above illustrates the relaxation exercise sequence, starting with shoulder rolls to release tension, proceeding with gentle neck stretches, and concluding with the arms floating above the head, swaying gently side to side, mimicking seaweed underwater. This scene captures the essence of tranquility and fluid motion, akin to being submerged in a peaceful, weightless underwater environment.

Day 3: Mindful Walking

- **Evening Activity (Duration: 15 minutes)**: Choose a safe, quiet place to walk, ideally in nature. As you walk, focus on the sensation of your feet making contact with the ground. Observe everything around you with a gentle curiosity. What do you see? What do you hear? How does the air feel?

Encouragement: This practice isn't about distance or speed; it's about being fully present with your walk. Let your thoughts come and go, returning your focus to the experience of walking.

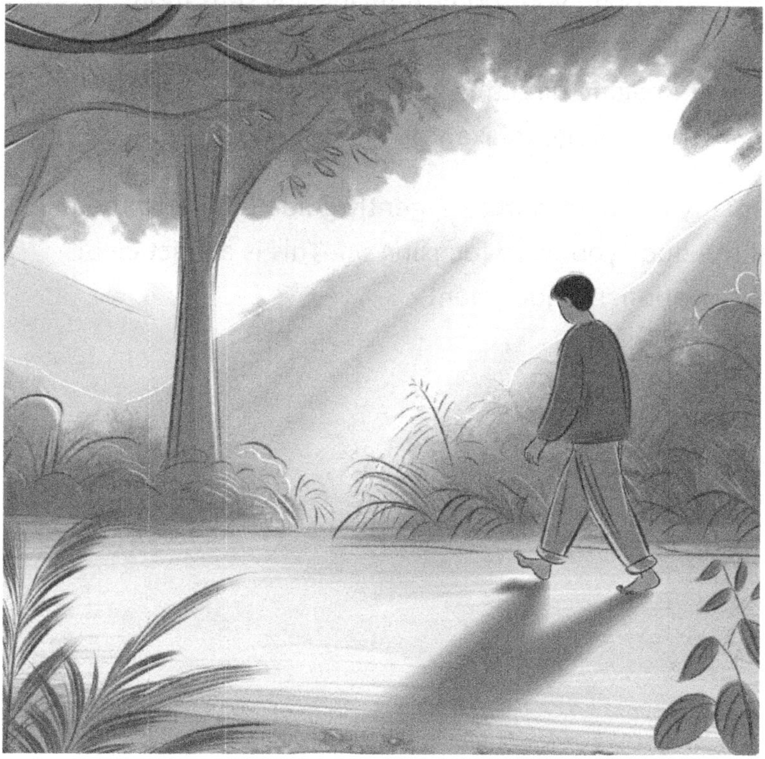

The image illustrates a peaceful walking scene in a natural setting, capturing the essence of mindfulness and connection with the earth. They convey the tranquility and serenity of walking in a quiet, natural area, focusing on the sensation of the feet making contact with the ground and observing the surroundings with gentle curiosity.

Day 4: Body Scan Meditation

- **Before Bed (Duration: 10-15 minutes)**: Lie down in a comfortable position, perhaps in bed or on a yoga mat, and close your eyes. Starting at the top of your head, slowly move your attention down through your body, noticing any sensations, tension, or relaxation. If you encounter tension, imagine directing your breath to that area to encourage relaxation.

Tip: If your mind wanders, gently guide it back to the part of the body you were focusing on. This is a practice of observation, not judgment.

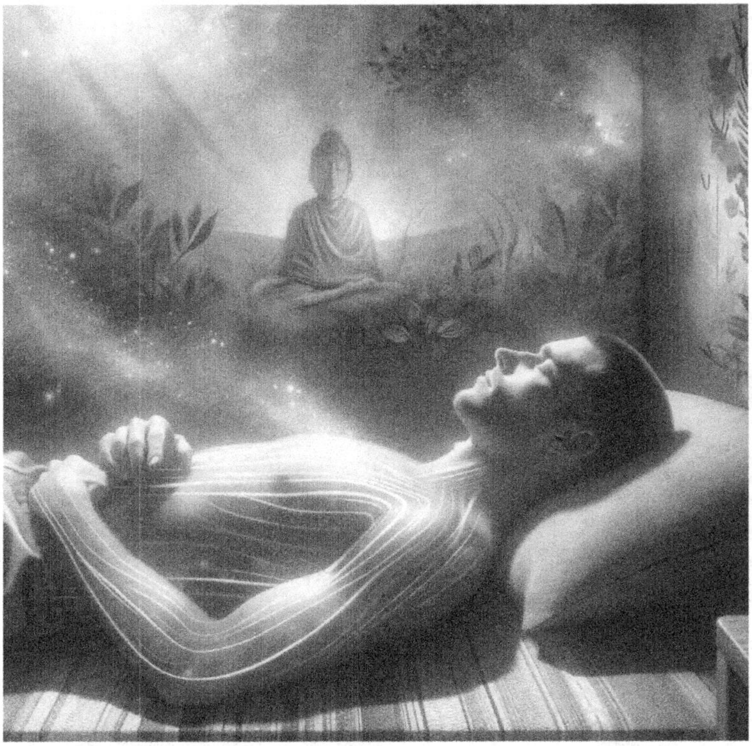

Here's the image depicting a peaceful and restorative scene, emphasizing the practice of mindfulness and body scan meditation as described.

Day 5: Expressive Movement

- **Fun Activity (Duration: 20 minutes)**: Create a playlist of your favorite songs that evoke different emotions. Play the music and allow your body to move however it wishes. This could be dancing, stretching, or even creating shapes with your body. Let the music guide you, and move in a way that expresses how you feel.

Adjustment: If you're not comfortable dancing, perhaps start with just moving your hands or swaying your body. The goal is to connect with your emotions through movement.

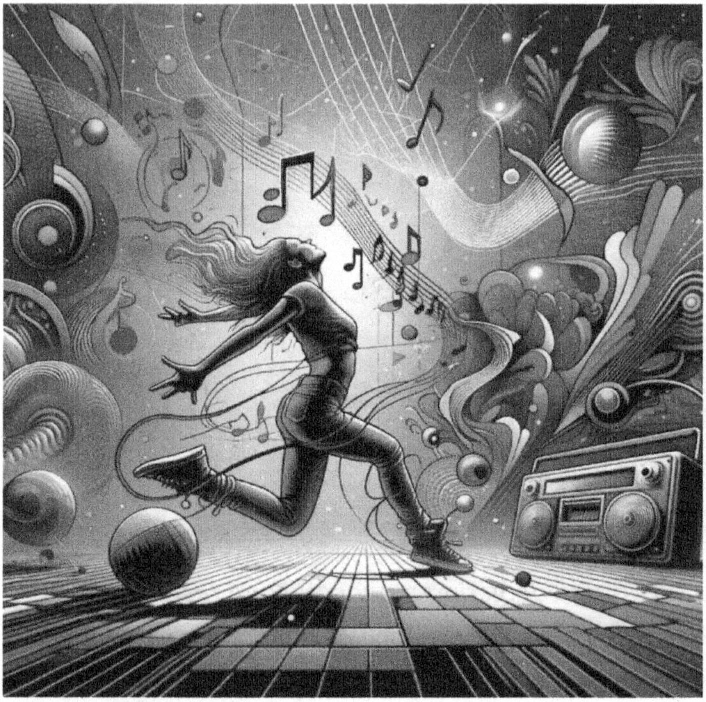

The image illustrates the dynamic and joyful expression of moving freely to music, capturing the essence of liberation and self-expression.

Day 6: Gratitude for Your Body

- **Reflection Time (Duration: 10 minutes)**: Find a quiet, comfortable space to sit. Close your eyes and take a few deep breaths. Think of three things you're grateful for about your body. It could be its ability to heal, the pleasure it brings you through taste, touch, or movement, or simply its resilience.

Encouragement: Practicing gratitude can shift your perspective from criticism to appreciation. This exercise is about recognizing the amazing capabilities of your body.

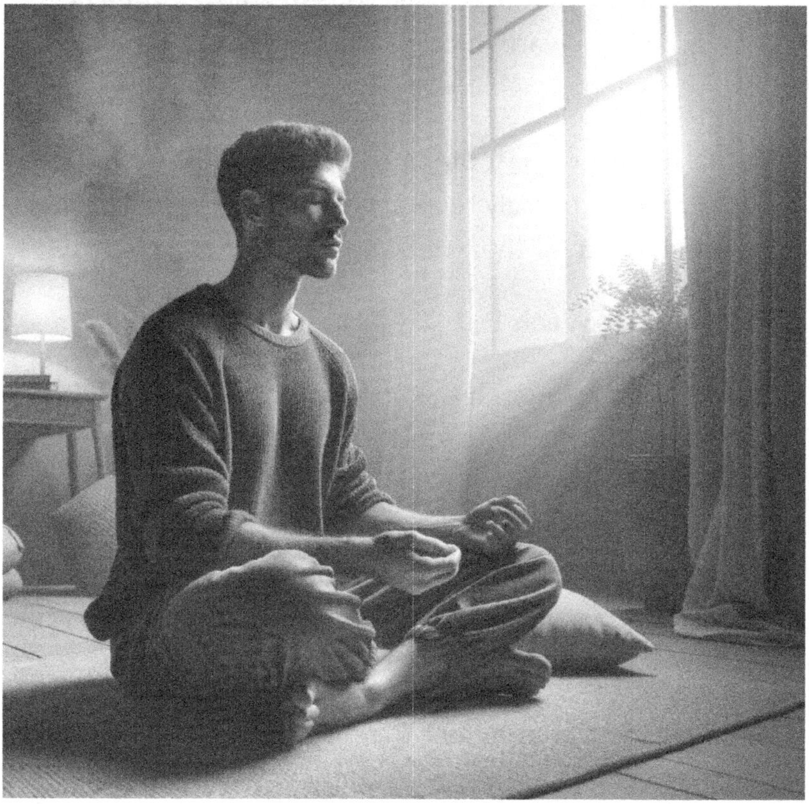

Day 7: Integrating and Resting

- **Self-Care Sunday (Duration: Flexible)**: Today is for rest and integration. Reflect on the week's activities and any insights you've gained about your body and its connection to your mind. Choose a restful activity that nourishes you—reading, journaling, taking a warm bath, or perhaps a gentle yoga session.

Tip: Rest is a vital part of the somatic wellness journey. Allow yourself to truly relax and recharge, preparing your body and mind for the week ahead.

Reflecting on Week 1

You've made it through the first week with wonderful dedication! How do you feel? Hopefully, you've started noticing a deeper connection with your body and a growing awareness of its signals. These daily activities are designed to be building blocks, laying the foundation for a more attuned and mindful relationship with your physical self.

As we progress, remember that these practices are flexible and meant to be adapted to your needs and responses. Your journey is unique, and how you engage with these exercises will evolve. Celebrate your commitment and curiosity—each step you take is a step toward greater wellness.

Mindfulness Practices for Setting Intentions and Cultivating Presence

Mindfulness practices are powerful tools for fostering a deeper connection with ourselves and the present moment. By setting intentions and cultivating presence, we can navigate our days with more awareness, purpose, and fulfillment. Let's explore some practices designed to help you set intentions and stay present, enhancing your overall well-being.

Setting Intentions with Mindfulness

1. Morning Intention Setting (Duration: 5 minutes)

- **Practice**: Start each day by sitting quietly in a comfortable space. Close your eyes and take a few deep breaths to center yourself. Ask, "What quality do I wish to bring into my day?" It could be kindness, patience, joy, or any other intention that resonates with you.
- **Implementation**: Visualize yourself embodying this quality in various situations throughout your day. Imagine how it feels, how you interact with others, and how others respond to you.
- **Tip**: Write your intention on a sticky note and place it where you'll see it throughout the day as a reminder to embody this quality.

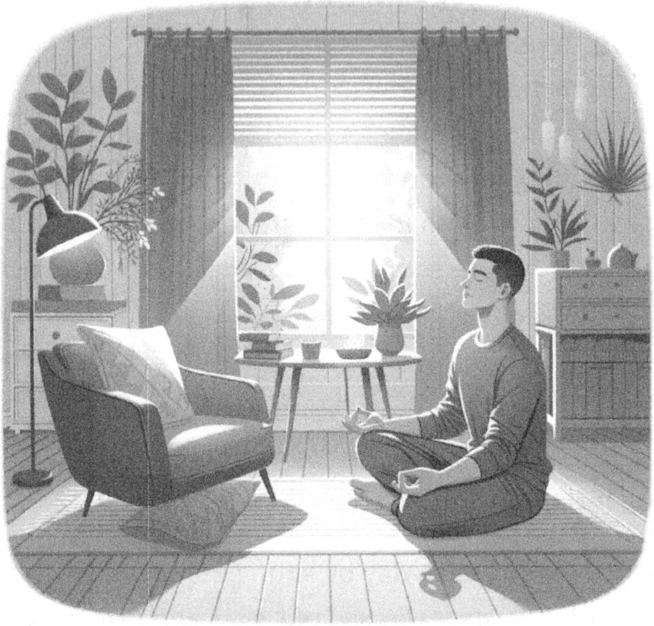

The image illustrates a peaceful morning routine, capturing the essence of starting the day with a moment of mindfulness and introspection in a serene setting.

2. Intentional Breathing Breaks (Duration: 2-3 minutes, multiple times a day)

- **Practice**: Set an alarm or reminder for several points during your day to pause for an intentional breathing break. Use this time to reconnect with your morning intention.
- **Implementation**: Take deep, slow breaths, focusing on your intention with each inhale and exhale. Let

this breathing ground you back into the present moment and your desired state of being.

- **Adjustment**: If your mind wanders, gently bring it back to your breath and intention. This is a practice of coming back to the moment and your chosen focus.

Cultivating Presence

3. Mindful Eating (Duration: At least one meal per day)

- **Practice**: Choose one meal or snack each day to eat mindfully. Before you begin, take a moment to express gratitude for the food. As you eat, pay attention to the flavors, textures, and sensations of eating, putting down your utensils between bites.
- **Implementation**: Notice the colors, smell, and even the sounds of your food. Chew slowly and savor each bite, fully engaging with the experience of eating.
- **Tip**: Try to eat without distractions like TV or reading. This practice is about fully immersing yourself in the act of eating and appreciating the nourishment your food provides.

4. Mindful Movement (Duration: 10-15 minutes daily)

- **Practice**: Incorporate a daily practice of mindful movement. This could be yoga, tai chi, walking, or simply stretching in a way that feels good to you.

- **Implementation**: As you move, focus your attention on how your body feels with each motion. Observe the sensations in your muscles and joints, and the rhythm of your breath.
- **Adjustment**: Adapt the movement to your body's needs on any given day. The goal is to be present with your body, not to achieve a specific form or intensity.

5. Daily Reflection (Duration: 5-10 minutes)

- **Practice**: End your day with a few minutes of reflection. Sit quietly and review your day with kindness and curiosity. Reflect on moments where you felt present and aligned with your intention, and moments where you were challenged.
- **Implementation**: Consider what you learned about yourself and how you might bring more presence and intention into your day tomorrow.
- **Tip**: Keep a journal of your reflections to track your progress and insights over time.

Integrating These Practices

By integrating these mindfulness practices into your daily routine, you're not just going through the motions of your day; you're living with intention and presence. This shift can transform your experience of life, making each moment richer and more meaningful. Remember, the journey of mindfulness is a personal one—there's no right or wrong way to practice. The key is consistency and a gentle, non-judgmental attitude toward yourself as you explore these practices.

Chapter 4: Week 2 - Building Strength and Flexibility

Progressive workouts for strength and flexibility

Progressive Exercises to Build Physical Strength and Increase Flexibility

Hey there! Ready to take the next step in building your physical strength and enhancing your flexibility? It's all about progressing at your own pace, listening to your body, and yes, having a bit of fun along the way. Let's dive into some exercises designed to help you grow stronger and more flexible, step by step.

Building Physical Strength

1. Bodyweight Squats (Duration: Start with 2 sets of 8-10 reps)

- **How to Do It**: Stand with your feet shoulder-width apart. Extend your arms straight out in front of you to help balance. Bend your knees and lower your body as if you're sitting back into a chair. Go down as far as comfortable, then push through your heels to return to standing.

- **Friendly Tip**: Imagine you're sitting down on an invisible chair. If going all the way down is tough, start by going halfway. It's all about improving over time!

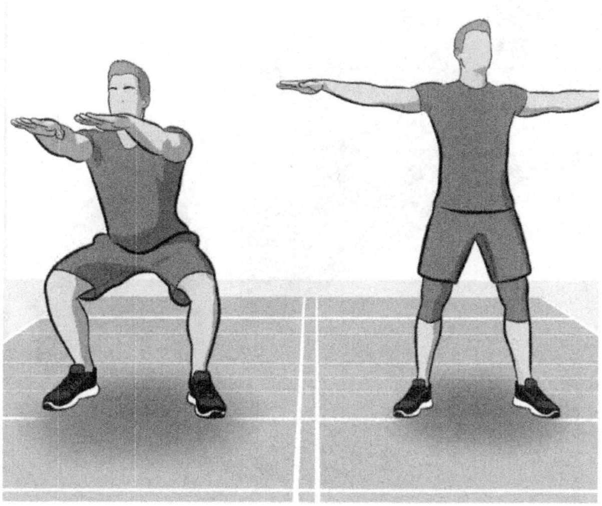

2. Push-ups (Duration: Start with 2 sets of 5-8 reps)

- **How to Do It**: Begin in a plank position with your hands slightly wider than your shoulders. Lower your body until your chest nearly touches the floor, elbows pointing back at a 45-degree angle, then push back up.
- **Adjustment**: If standard push-ups are challenging, start with your knees on the ground. You're still building strength, and that's awesome!

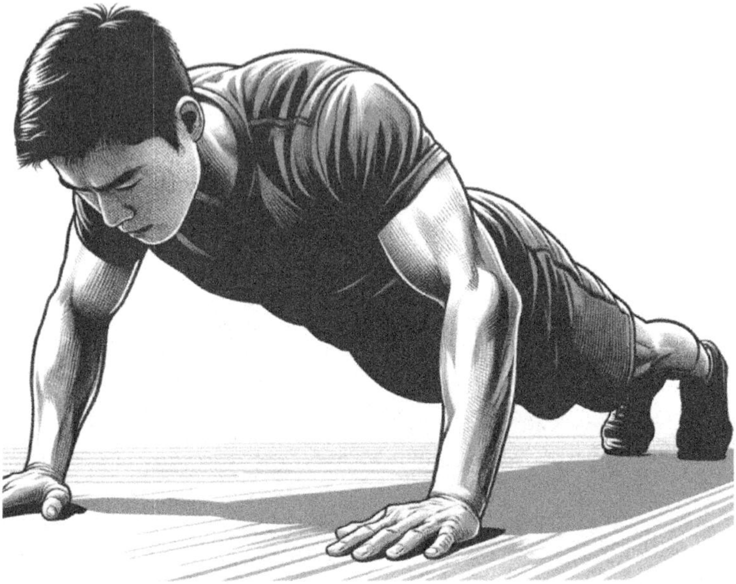

3. Plank (Duration: Start with 2 sets of 20-30 seconds)

- **How to Do It**: Support your body on your toes and forearms with your elbows directly under your shoulders. Keep your body in a straight line from head to heels.
- **Encouragement**: Planks are tough but super effective. If you need to start with shorter durations, that's totally okay. Every second counts, and you're doing great!

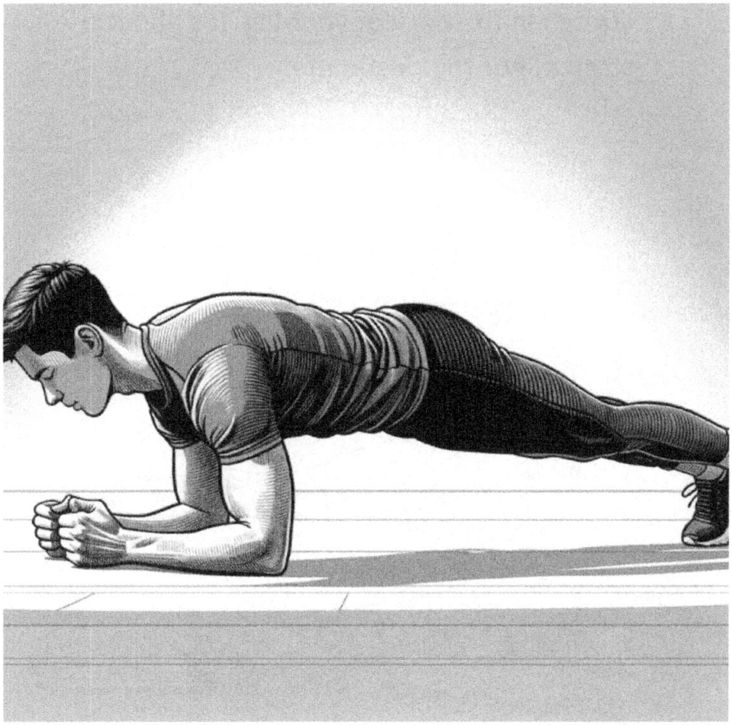

Increasing Flexibility

1. Hamstring Stretch (Duration: Hold for 20-30 seconds each leg)

- **How to Do It**: Sit on the floor with one leg extended and the other bent, foot resting against the opposite inner thigh. Reach toward the toes of your extended leg, keeping your knee as straight as comfortable. Switch legs and repeat.
- **Friendly Tip**: Don't worry if you can't touch your toes. Just reach forward gently until you feel a

stretch in the back of your leg. It's about the stretch, not the destination.

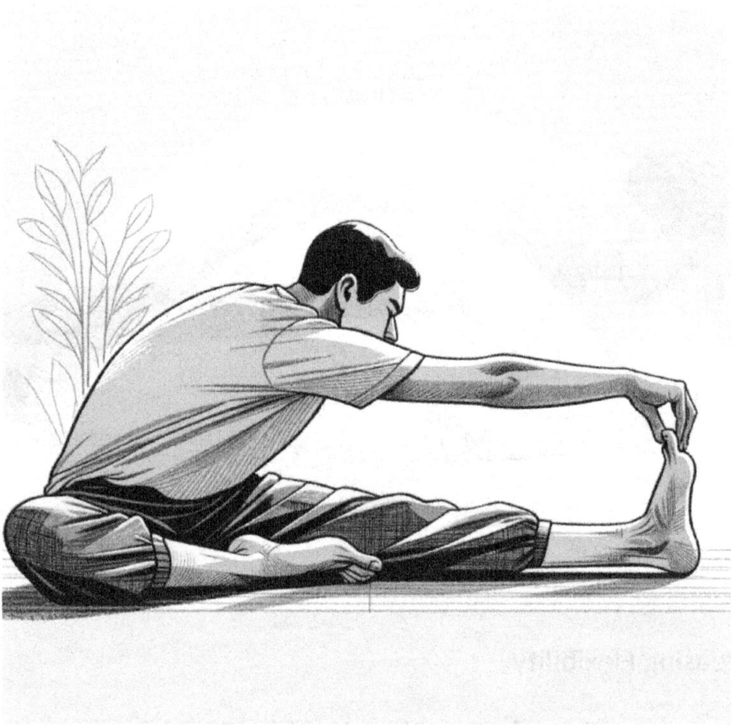

2. Cat-Cow Stretch (Duration: 1-2 minutes, flowing between poses)

- **How to Do It**: Start on your hands and knees in a tabletop position. Inhale as you arch your back, tilting your pelvis and head upward (Cow). Exhale as you round your back, tucking your chin to your chest and pulling your belly in (Cat).

- **Encouragement**: This exercise is great for spinal flexibility. Feel free to linger in positions that feel especially good. Listen to your body—it knows what it needs.

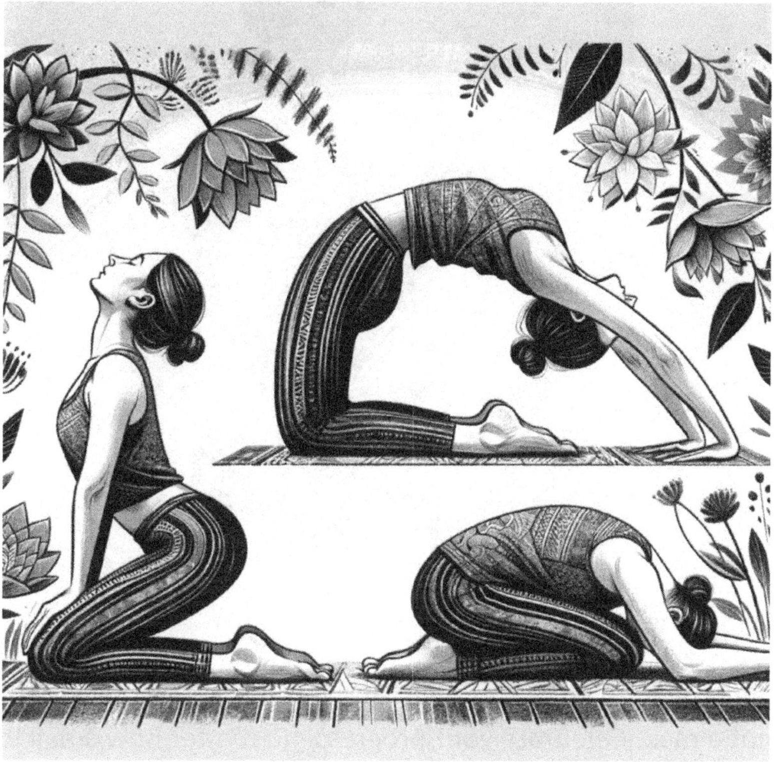

3. Chest Opener (Duration: Hold for 20-30 seconds)

- **How to Do It**: Stand or sit upright and clasp your hands behind your back. Gently straighten your arms and lift them slightly, opening up your chest.
- **Adjustment**: If clasping your hands is tricky, hold a towel between them to help bridge the gap. You're opening your chest and heart to the world—how cool is that?

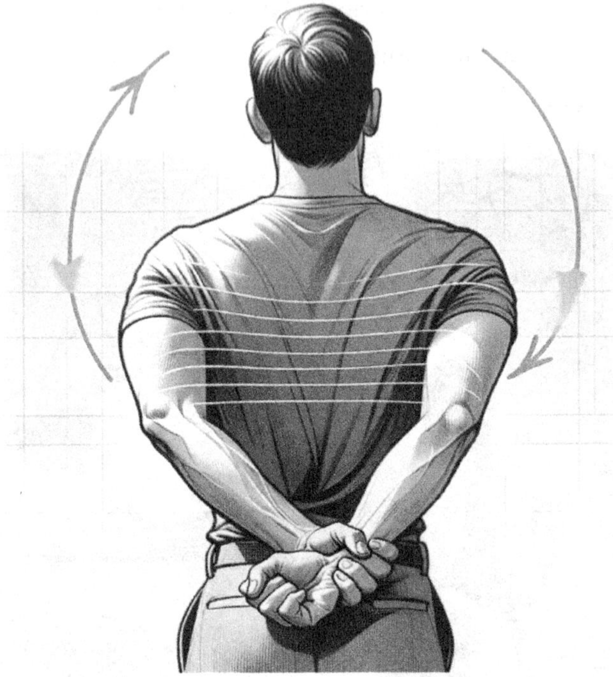

Wrapping Up

Remember, building strength and flexibility is a journey, not a race. Celebrate your progress, no matter how small it may seem. Every rep, every stretch, every moment you dedicate to your health is a victory. Be patient and kind to yourself, and don't hesitate to adjust these exercises to fit your needs. You're doing an amazing job, and I'm here cheering you on every step of the way. Let's keep this positive momentum going!

Integrating Mindfulness into Physical Activity

Hey! Ready to blend mindfulness with your physical activities? It's like adding a dash of spice to your favorite dish—it enhances the whole experience. Integrating mindfulness means paying close attention to our bodies, our movements, and the present moment, turning exercise from routine to a rich, engaging experience. Let's dive into some techniques that can help you get there, with plenty of room for personal tweaks.

Mindful Walking or Running

How to Do It: Whether you're walking or running, focus on your breath and the sensation of your feet touching the ground. Notice the rhythm of your steps and how your arms swing with each stride.

Friendly Tip: Every few minutes, check in with your body. How are your shoulders feeling? Can you relax them a bit more? Are you clenching your jaw? Let it loosen. This isn't just about moving from point A to B; it's about really experiencing the journey.

Adjustment: If your mind starts to wander, gently bring it back to the sensation of movement or your breath. It's normal for thoughts to drift, and the practice is in the returning, not staying perfectly focused.

Mindful Strength Training

How to Do It: When lifting weights or doing bodyweight exercises, concentrate on the muscle groups you're engaging. Feel the muscles contract and relax with each movement. Pay attention to your form and the smooth flow of motion.

Encouragement: Celebrate the effort your body is putting in, even if you're starting with lighter weights or fewer reps. It's about the quality of each movement, not just the quantity.

Friendly Tip: Before you start each set, take a deep breath and set an intention for that specific exercise. Maybe it's to stay fully present or to appreciate your body's strength. Let this intention guide your focus.

Mindful Yoga or Stretching

How to Do It: As you move into each pose or stretch, focus on the sensations in your body. Notice areas of tension and areas of ease. Breathe into any tightness, imagining each exhale creating a little more space in your body.

Adjustment: Yoga and stretching are perfect for exploring mindfulness, as they naturally encourage attention to breath and body. If a pose doesn't feel right, modify it. This is your practice, and it's all about listening to your body.

Friendly Tip: Use the transitions between poses to maintain mindfulness. How does it feel to move from one pose to another? Can you find grace and awareness in the movement itself?

Integrating Breathwork

How to Do It: During any physical activity, bring your attention to your breath. Try to synchronize your movements with your breathing—for example, inhale as you lift a weight, and exhale as you lower it.

Encouragement: If coordinating breath and movement feels tricky, no worries! Just bringing your attention back to your breath is a fantastic start. Over time, this synchronization can become a powerful tool for deepening mindfulness in motion.

Wrapping It Up

Merging mindfulness with physical activity can transform your workouts from something you "have to do" into something you're deeply engaged in and enjoy. It turns exercise into a practice of self-care and awareness, where every breath and movement is an opportunity to connect with the present moment.

Remember, there's no "perfect" way to be mindful. It's all about exploration, curiosity, and finding what works best for you. So go ahead, give these techniques a try, and see how they change your exercise experience. Here's to moving mindfully and discovering the joy in every step, lift, and stretch!

Real-Life Examples of Integrating Mindfulness into Physical Activity

Let's bring the concept of mindfulness in physical activity to life with some real-life examples. These stories highlight how everyday people, perhaps someone just like you, have woven mindfulness into their exercise routines, transforming their experiences and deepening their connection to their bodies.

Emma's Mindful Running Journey

Emma used to view running as just a way to stay in shape. It was more of a chore than a pleasure, until she decided to try mindful running. Instead of blasting music or zoning out during her runs, she started focusing on her breath, the rhythm of her feet hitting the pavement, and the sensations in her body. She noticed the colors of the sky, the sound of the birds, and the changing scenery around her. This shift didn't just make running more enjoyable; it became a moving meditation. Emma found that her runs left her feeling more grounded and peaceful, transforming her relationship with running from a must-do exercise to a cherished practice.

Yoga with Mark: A Journey of Awareness

Mark was always into fitness, but he approached yoga purely as a physical workout. That changed when he joined a class that emphasized the mindfulness aspect of yoga. Instead of rushing through poses, he began to slow down, paying attention to his breath and how each movement felt in his body. This mindful approach helped him notice when he was pushing too hard and when he could gently extend his limits. Yoga became a space for Mark to explore his physical and mental edges, teaching him patience and self-compassion, and bringing a sense of calm and balance into his life.

Lily's Strength Training Transformation

Lily started strength training to build muscle and improve her health. Initially focused on lifting as much weight as possible, she often ended her sessions feeling drained and occasionally injured. After learning about mindful exercise, Lily shifted her approach. She began to concentrate on her breathing and the muscles she was working, taking the time to feel each movement and its impact on her body. This not only improved her form and reduced injuries but also made her more aware of her body's capabilities and limits. Lily's workouts became more effective and enjoyable, transforming her time in the gym into an empowering practice of self-awareness and strength.

The Peaceful Swimmer: Sarah's Story

Sarah swam laps for exercise, usually counting laps to pass the time. After incorporating mindfulness into her swimming, she started focusing on the sensation of the water against her skin, the rhythm of her stroke and breath, and the quiet underwater sounds. This shift made her aware of a profound sense of peace and fluidity in her movements. Swimming became a time for Sarah to clear her mind and immerse herself in the present moment, enhancing both her physical and mental well-being.

The Takeaway

These stories show that mindfulness can transform any physical activity into a more meaningful and enriching experience. Whether running, yoga, strength training, or swimming, bringing attention to the present moment deepens our connection to our activities and ourselves. Emma, Mark, Lily, and Sarah discovered that mindfulness in motion not only enhances physical performance but also nurtures mental and emotional health, proving that the journey is just as important as the destination. Let their stories inspire you to explore mindfulness in your physical activities and discover the depth and richness it can add to your own experience.

Chapter 5: Week 3 - Enhancing Emotional Balance

Emotional awareness through somatic practices

Integrating somatic awareness into the process of identifying, expressing, and managing emotions can transform your relationship with your feelings, leading to deeper understanding and healthier emotional regulation. Somatic practices focus on the body's sensations and movements, offering a powerful pathway to connect with and navigate your emotional landscape. Here are some exercises and practices designed to help you engage with your emotions somatically.

1. Body Scan for Emotional Awareness

Practice: Begin with a body scan to identify how your emotions manifest physically. Find a comfortable, quiet space to sit or lie down. Close your eyes, take a few deep breaths, and gradually direct your attention through different parts of your body. Notice any sensations—tightness, warmth, tingling, or anything else.

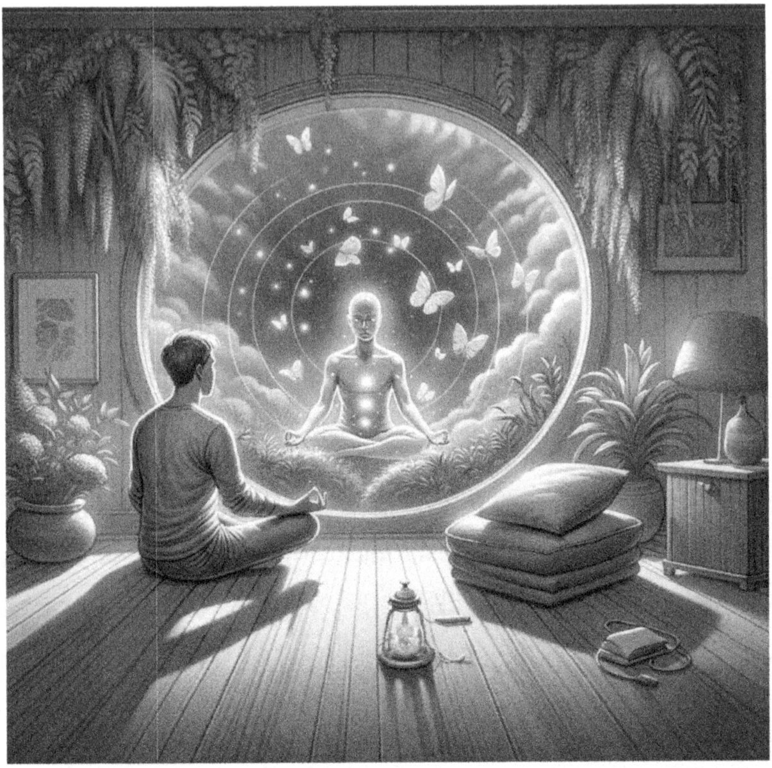

The image visualizes a tranquil scene of engaging in a body scan meditation, focusing on the connection between emotions and their physical manifestations within a serene and introspective setting.

Application: As you notice these sensations, ask yourself what emotions might be connected to them. For example, a tight chest might be associated with anxiety, while a heavy stomach might relate to sadness. This practice helps you link physical sensations to emotional states.

Friendly Tip: Remember, there's no right or wrong here. Whatever you feel is valid and worth exploring.

2. Grounding Techniques for Emotional Regulation

Practice: Grounding techniques can help stabilize your emotions by bringing your focus back to the present moment. One effective method is the "5-4-3-2-1" technique, where you identify:

- 5 things you can see,
- 4 things you can touch,
- 3 things you can hear,
- 2 things you can smell, and
- 1 thing you can taste.

Application: Use this technique when you feel overwhelmed by emotions. It can help interrupt spiraling thoughts and bring you back to the here and now.

Adjustment: If you're in a place where some senses can't be engaged, focus more on those you can. The key is to connect with your immediate environment.

3. Expressive Movement to Release Emotions

Practice: Sometimes, emotions are too complex to articulate with words. In such times, expressive movement can be a powerful outlet. Put on some music that resonates with your current emotional state, and allow your body to move freely, without judgment or preconception.

Application: Let your movements express what you're feeling. You might find yourself dancing, stretching, or even curling up and uncurling. This practice can help release stored emotions in your body and can be incredibly liberating.

Friendly Tip: There's no audience here, and there's no "right" way to move. Trust your body and let it lead the way.

4. Breathwork for Emotional Management

Practice: Breathwork can significantly impact your emotional state. Try the 4-7-8 breathing technique to calm anxiety or stress. Breathe in through your nose for 4 seconds, hold your breath for 7 seconds, and exhale slowly through your mouth for 8 seconds.

Application: Use this breathing pattern whenever you feel anxious or upset. It helps regulate the nervous system and can bring a sense of calm and control.

Adjustment: If holding your breath for 7 seconds is uncomfortable, adjust the numbers as needed. The extended exhale is the key component here.

5. Journaling for Emotional Clarity

Practice: After engaging in somatic practices, take some time to journal about your experiences. Write down what emotions surfaced, where you felt them in your body, and any thoughts or memories that came up.

Application: This practice can help you process your emotions more deeply and gain insights into your emotional patterns and triggers.

Friendly Tip: Try to write without editing yourself. Let your thoughts and feelings flow freely. This is for your eyes only.

6. Somatic "Check-Ins" Throughout the Day

Practice: Set a few reminders on your phone or watch to pause for a quick somatic "check-in" with yourself throughout the day. This involves pausing whatever you're doing, taking a deep breath, and noticing any sensations in your body.

Application: Ask yourself, "What am I feeling right now, and where do I feel it in my body?" This practice helps you become more aware of how emotions ebb and flow throughout the day, and how they manifest physically.

Friendly Tip: If you identify any discomfort or tension, acknowledge it without judgment. Consider what might be needed in that moment—perhaps a stretch, a walk, or a few deep breaths.

7. Progressive Muscle Relaxation for Emotional Release

Practice: Progressive muscle relaxation involves tensing and then relaxing different muscle groups in your body. This can be particularly effective for releasing emotional tension.

Application: Start from the top of your head and work down to your toes, tensing each muscle group for a few seconds, then releasing. Pay special attention to areas where you commonly hold stress, such as your jaw, shoulders, or stomach.

Adjustment: If you find it hard to tense and relax specific muscle groups, focus on deep breathing instead, imagining tension leaving your body with each exhale.

8. Emotional Grounding Through Nature Connection

Practice: Spending time in nature is a powerful way to ground yourself and connect with your emotions somatically. Whether it's a walk in the park, gardening, or simply sitting under a tree, nature can help soothe and reset your emotional state.

Application: Try to engage all your senses while in nature. Notice the colors, smells, sounds, and the feel of the air or ground. This multisensory approach can help anchor you in the present moment and provide a calm backdrop for emotional processing.

Friendly Tip: If you can't get outside, even looking at nature images or listening to nature sounds can have a calming effect.

9. Dancing to Express and Process Emotions

Practice: Dancing is a dynamic way to express emotions that might be hard to put into words. It combines physical movement, creativity, and emotional release.

Application: Put on music that resonates with how you're feeling, and let your body move freely, without worrying about how it looks. Allow your emotions to guide your movements, using dance as a form of emotional storytelling.

Friendly Tip: Closing your eyes might help you focus inward and enhance the emotional expression through movement.

10. Partnered Somatic Practices for Shared Emotional Support

Practice: Engaging in somatic practices with a partner, such as synchronized breathing, partner yoga, or even just holding hands and sharing a moment of silence, can create a shared space for emotional support and connection.

Application: With a trusted friend or partner, try sitting back-to-back, focusing on breathing in sync for a few minutes. Share any emotions or sensations that arise without judgment.

Friendly Tip: Communication is key. Make sure both partners feel safe and comfortable sharing this space and are open to discussing their experiences afterward.

Bringing It All Together

These somatic practices offer diverse ways to explore and manage your emotions through body awareness. Whether you're engaging in a solo practice like progressive muscle relaxation or sharing a somatic experience with a partner, the goal is to deepen your connection to your emotional self in a healthy, embodied way. Remember, integrating these practices into your life is a journey. Be patient and compassionate with yourself as you explore what works best for you, and celebrate the steps you take towards emotional wellness and somatic awareness.

Somatic practices for emotional resilience

Enhancing Emotional Resilience Through Somatic Practices

Building emotional resilience isn't about avoiding feelings; it's about navigating through them with grace and strength. Somatic practices offer a pathway to achieving this by helping you tune into your body's wisdom. Let's explore some strategies and exercises that can bolster your emotional resilience, all while keeping it light, personal, and exploratory.

1. Anchoring in the Breath

Strategy: Your breath is a powerful tool for regulating emotions. By learning to control and focus on your breath, you can calm your nervous system and gain perspective in stressful situations.

Practice: Try the 4-7-8 breathing technique whenever you feel overwhelmed. Breathe in for 4 seconds, hold for 7, and exhale for 8. This helps activate your parasympathetic nervous system, the part of your body that signals relaxation.

Friendly Tip: If the 4-7-8 count feels too long, adjust it to what feels comfortable. The key is the prolonged exhale, which helps calm the mind.

2. Grounding Through the Senses

Strategy: Grounding can bring you back to the present moment, reducing anxiety and stress. It's about reconnecting with the here and now, using your senses as guides.

Practice: Engage in a sensory walk, either outside or even in your home. Focus on one sense at a time—what you can see, hear, smell, touch, and taste. Allow these sensory experiences to anchor you in the present.

Friendly Tip: If you're indoors and limited with sensory options, try focusing on textures around you or the taste of a piece of fruit. It's all about noticing the small details.

3. Releasing Stored Emotions Through Movement

Strategy: Emotions can get stored in our bodies as tension. Using movement intentionally can help release this tension and the emotions tied to it.

Practice: Set aside time to move in a way that feels releasing for you. This could be dancing, shaking (literally shaking off stress), or even a vigorous workout. Pay attention to areas of tension and imagine sending breath and movement to those spots.

Friendly Tip: If you're not sure where to start, begin with shaking out each limb individually, then progress to your whole body. Notice how even a few minutes of this can change how you feel.

4. Cultivating Body Awareness and Compassion

Strategy: Developing a compassionate relationship with your body enhances emotional resilience by fostering self-acceptance and understanding.

Practice: Practice a daily body scan meditation, focusing on sending gratitude and kindness to each part of your body. Acknowledge the work your body does for you every day, and offer it your compassion.

Adjustment: If sitting still for a meditation is challenging, try doing a body scan while lying down before sleep, blending relaxation with gratitude.

5. Creating a Somatic Resource Bank

Strategy: A somatic resource bank is a collection of physical sensations, movements, or memories that evoke feelings of safety, joy, or calm. These can be drawn upon in times of stress.

Practice: Reflect on activities or memories that bring you a sense of peace. It could be the feeling of sun on your skin, the sound of laughter, or a comforting hug. Practice recalling these sensations in detail, anchoring them in your body.

Friendly Tip: Keep a journal of these resources. When you're feeling low, revisit your bank and choose a resource to focus on, bringing those good sensations back into the present moment.

Wrapping It Up

Building emotional resilience is a journey, and it's uniquely yours. By incorporating these somatic practices into your life, you're not just reacting to emotions as they come; you're actively crafting a more resilient and responsive emotional landscape. Remember, exploration and curiosity are your best friends here. Adjust, adapt, and align these practices with what feels right for you. Celebrate each step you take towards resilience, knowing that with each practice, you're nurturing a stronger, more connected self.

Chapter 6: Week 4 - Integrating Somatic Wellness into Daily Life

Sustaining Somatic Wellness After 30 Days: Advanced Techniques

Sustaining Somatic Wellness: Advanced Techniques

So, you've made it through the initial 30 days of integrating somatic practices into your life—congratulations! Now, let's talk about how to sustain and deepen these practices long-term. It's all about making this journey enjoyable, meaningful, and uniquely yours. Ready to explore some advanced techniques? Let's dive in.

1. Intuitive Movement

Advanced Technique: This involves listening deeply to your body's needs and responding with movement that feels nourishing and right in the moment, without following a specific routine or plan.

Practice: Start by standing still and taking a few deep breaths. Then, allow your body to move in any way it wants. It might be slow stretching, dynamic dancing, or anything in between. The key is to let your body lead, turning off the mind's chatter.

Friendly Tip: If you find yourself thinking, "Am I doing this right?" gently remind yourself that there's no right or wrong here. This practice is about connecting with your body's wisdom.

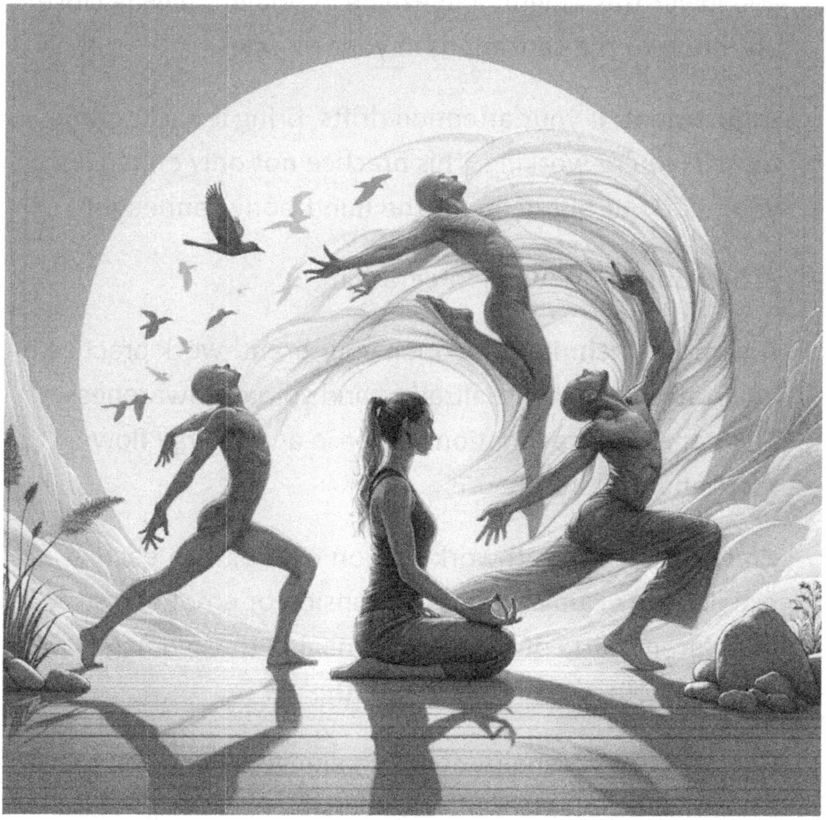

2. Mindful Resistance Training

Advanced Technique: Incorporate mindfulness into strength training by focusing intensely on the muscle groups you're working. Notice the sensation of muscle contraction and release, and align your breath with your movements.

Practice: For example, when doing a bicep curl, focus on the feeling of your bicep muscles as they work. Inhale as you lower the weight, and exhale as you lift, paying close attention to the sensations in your muscles.

Adjustment: If your attention drifts, bring it back to the muscle you're working. This practice not only enhances your workout but deepens the mind-body connection.

3. Somatic Breathwork Integration

Advanced Technique: Deepen your breathwork practice by integrating it with visualization and somatic awareness. This can enhance emotional release and energy flow throughout the body.

Practice: Try a breathwork session where, with each exhale, you visualize releasing tension or emotions stored in different parts of your body. Imagine these being breathed out and dissolved into the air.

Friendly Tip: If visualization is challenging, focus on the sensation of release with each exhale. Feel the physical letting go in your body, which can be just as powerful.

4. Eco-Somatics: Connecting with Nature

Advanced Technique: This practice involves deepening your somatic awareness through direct interaction with nature, using its elements to foster a deeper connection with your body and the earth.

Practice: Spend time in nature, and choose an element (earth, water, air, or fire) to focus on. For example, feel the earth under your feet, notice the air on your skin, listen to the sound of water, or watch the movement of flames in a campfire. Reflect on how this element feels in your body and what emotions or sensations arise.

Friendly Tip: If you can't be outside, use natural elements like a bowl of water or a stone to connect with these sensations indoors.

5. Somatic Journaling

Advanced Technique: After engaging in somatic practices, take time to journal about your experiences. This can help integrate and deepen your understanding of your body's signals and the emotional landscape within.

Practice: Write about what you noticed in your body during the practice, any emotions that surfaced, and any insights or thoughts that came up. Over time, you'll create a rich map of your somatic experiences.

Friendly Tip: Don't worry about grammar or making it "perfect." This journal is a tool for exploration and reflection, just for you.

6. Partner Somatic Exercises

Advanced Technique: Engaging in somatic practices with a partner can enhance your awareness and introduce new dimensions of connection and support.

Practice: Try a simple mirroring exercise where you and your partner mimic each other's movements in a slow, intentional manner. Focus on the sensation of movement and the subtle non-verbal communication happening between you.

Friendly Tip: Maintain eye contact if comfortable, as it can deepen the connection. Remember, this is a conversation without words, a chance to explore empathy and connectedness through movement.

7. Somatic Meditation in Motion

Advanced Technique: Combine meditation with movement to cultivate a deeply meditative state while engaging your body. This can be a walking meditation, tai chi, or even a slow, mindful yoga practice where the focus is on inner sensations and breath.

Practice: Choose a form of gentle movement that you enjoy. As you move, direct your focus inward. Observe the sensations in your body, the flow of your breath, and any emotions or thoughts that arise, letting them pass without attachment.

Adjustment: If your mind wanders, gently guide it back to your body's sensations or your breath. This practice is about being present in each moment, each movement.

8. Somatic Visualization Techniques

Advanced Technique: Visualization can powerfully enhance somatic awareness, helping you connect with and shift your body's energy.

Practice: While in a relaxed state, visualize a warm, healing light moving through your body. Imagine this light soothing tensions, dissolving blockages, and energizing every cell. Focus on areas that may need extra attention, and allow yourself to feel the sensations this visualization brings.

Friendly Tip: Use this technique as a way to start or end your day, or even as a quick midday reset. It's a gentle yet powerful way to realign your body and mind.

9. Exploring Somatic Creativity

Advanced Technique: Creativity and somatics go hand in hand. Use creative expression as a way to explore and communicate your somatic experiences.

Practice: After a somatic exercise, grab some art supplies and create something that represents your experience. This could be a drawing, painting, or even a poem. Don't worry about artistic skill; focus on expressing what you felt in your body.

Friendly Tip: This practice can unlock new insights about your somatic journey and provide a visual or written record of your growth and discoveries.

10. Somatic Listening and Dialogue

Advanced Technique: Develop a practice of "somatic listening" to deepen your understanding of your body's signals and messages.

Practice: Spend a few moments each day sitting quietly, asking your body what it needs or wants to communicate. Listen without judgment. You might receive answers in the form of sensations, emotions, or even intuitive thoughts.

Friendly Tip: Keep a journal specifically for this practice. Over time, you'll develop a deeper dialogue with your body, uncovering insights and guidance from within.

Embracing Lifelong Somatic Exploration

Your somatic wellness journey is unique and ever-evolving. By incorporating these advanced techniques, you're not just maintaining your practice; you're expanding it, exploring the rich tapestry of connections between your body, mind, and the world around you. Remember, somatic wellness is not a destination but a way of living—a continuous exploration of how to be fully present and alive in your body. Keep exploring, stay curious, and celebrate each discovery as a step toward deeper wellness and harmony.

Crafting Your Personalized, Adaptable Somatic Routine

Hey there! Creating a somatic routine that's tailored just for you is like designing your own personal wellness journey. This isn't about following a strict regimen but about finding what feels good and what resonates with your body and emotions day by day. Let's walk through how to build this flexible, joyful practice together.

1. Start with Intention

Set Your Intention: Begin by asking yourself what you hope to achieve with your somatic practice. Is it stress relief? Enhanced body awareness? Emotional balance? This intention will be your guiding star.

Friendly Tip: Your intention can change, and that's perfectly okay! Check in with yourself regularly to see if your goals are evolving.

2. Mix and Match Practices

Choose Your Elements: Think of your somatic routine as a mix-and-match menu. Include elements of movement (like yoga or dancing), mindfulness (meditation or breathwork), and restorative practices (body scans or progressive muscle relaxation).

Try This: Don't feel like you have to stick to the same activities every day. One day you might need more vigorous movement, and another, more gentle stretching or meditation. Listen to your body's needs.

3. Schedule Flexibly

Find Your Time: Identify times in your day when you can realistically integrate these practices. Morning might work for some, while others might find evening routines more beneficial.

Adjustment: If your schedule is unpredictable, that's okay! Even five minutes of deep breathing or a quick body scan can be incredibly beneficial. It's about quality, not quantity.

4. Tune Into Your Body

Body Check-In: Before each practice, do a quick check-in with your body. How are you feeling physically? Emotionally? Let this check-in inform your practice choice for the day.

Friendly Tip: Some days you might find certain areas of tension or discomfort. Use this information to choose practices that address these sensations directly.

5. Keep It Dynamic

Change It Up: Allow your routine to evolve. Try new somatic exercises or practices as you discover them. Keeping your routine dynamic helps maintain your interest and engagement over time.

Try This: Every couple of weeks, swap out one of your routine elements for something new. It could be a different style of meditation, a new movement practice, or even exploring nature walks.

6. Reflect and Adjust

Journaling: After your practice, spend a few minutes reflecting on the experience. What worked well? What didn't? How do you feel now compared to before?

Friendly Tip: Use this reflection to tweak your routine. Maybe you discover that you prefer longer meditation sessions or that certain movements are especially rewarding. This reflection is key to personalization.

7. Cultivate a Supportive Environment

Create Your Space: If possible, dedicate a space in your home for your somatic practices. This doesn't have to be an entire room—a corner or a specific chair can work just as well.

Adjustment: If space is limited, consider how to quickly transform a part of your living area into your practice space with a mat, a cushion, or even just a specific blanket.

Bringing It All Together

Your somatic routine is deeply personal and should reflect your individual needs, preferences, and lifestyle. It's all about exploration and adaptation. Remember, the goal is to build a practice that feels refreshing, supportive, and aligned with your journey towards wellness. There's no "right" way to do this—only what's right for you. Celebrate your commitment to self-awareness and somatic wellness, and enjoy the journey of discovering what makes you feel most alive and connected.

Part III: Deepening Your Practice

Chapter 7: Overcoming Common Challenges

Overcoming Common Challenges

Navigating the Roadblocks on Your Somatic Journey

Hey, it's completely normal to hit some bumps along the way in your journey towards somatic wellness. Whether it's finding the time, sparking up motivation, or feeling like you're not making progress, these challenges don't define your journey—they're just part of it. Let's talk through these, one by one, with some kindness and practical advice, like a good friend would.

When Time Feels Scarce

It's tough trying to fit in wellness practices when your schedule is packed, right? The key here is not the length of time you dedicate, but the consistency and quality of that time.

Practical Advice: Start small. Even five minutes of deep breathing or a quick body scan can make a big difference. Try integrating somatic practices into activities you're already doing—mindful breathing while waiting for your coffee to brew, or a few stretches during a break at work. Remember, this is about weaving wellness into your life, not adding another hefty task to your to-do list.

Sparking Motivation

Some days, the drive just isn't there, and that's okay. Motivation ebbs and flows, and sometimes we need to find external sources to help reignite it.

Practical Advice: Set up reminders of why you started this journey. It could be a note on your mirror, a daily alarm with a motivational quote, or even a photo that reminds you of your goals. Also, consider a wellness buddy. Sharing your journey with someone can boost your motivation, especially on days when it's lagging. Lastly, celebrate every little win, no matter how small it seems. Acknowledging your efforts can be a powerful motivator.

Feeling Stuck or Not Seeing Progress

It can be disheartening when you feel like you're not moving forward. Remember, progress in somatic practices isn't always linear or measurable in the traditional sense. It's about deepening your connection with yourself, which can be subtle.

Practical Advice: Shift your focus from outcomes to experiences. Notice how you feel during and after your practices. Are you a bit calmer, more present, or maybe just a little kinder to yourself? That's progress. Also, try journaling your experiences. Over time, you'll likely see shifts you hadn't noticed day-to-day. And don't be afraid to switch things up. Sometimes, trying a new practice can reignite your enthusiasm and open up new avenues of growth.

When Routine Becomes Monotonous

Sometimes, even the most fulfilling practices can start to feel stale. It's normal. The beauty of somatic wellness lies in its vast landscape of practices you can explore.

Practical Advice: Shake things up! If you've been focusing on one type of practice, why not explore another? If yoga has been your go-to, try integrating dynamic dance movements or tai chi. Alternatively, switch environments. If you usually practice indoors, take your practice outside to a park or your backyard. Fresh scenery can bring fresh energy to your routine.

Overcoming Self-Judgment

It's easy to be your own harshest critic, especially when progress seems slow or when you compare your journey with others'. Remember, somatic wellness is deeply personal, and there's no standard timeline or comparison chart.

Practical Advice: Practice self-compassion. Speak to yourself as you would to a dear friend—kindly, empathetically, and encouragingly. Recognize your efforts, no matter how small they seem. Every moment you dedicate to this journey is a step forward. Affirmations can be powerful tools here. Try starting your day by affirming, "I am on my own unique path, and I am exactly where I need to be."

When Doubt Creeps In

Doubt is a natural part of any journey, especially one as introspective as somatic wellness. It's okay to have moments of doubt; what's important is how you navigate them.

Practical Advice: Connect with your 'why.' Revisit the reasons you started this journey. Reflecting on your initial intentions can reignite your passion and clear away doubts. Additionally, engaging with a community—whether online or in person—can provide support and reassurance. Hearing others' experiences and sharing your own can be incredibly affirming.

Finding Balance Between Effort and Ease

In somatic practices, there's a delicate balance between pushing yourself and allowing yourself to rest. Finding this balance is key to a sustainable practice.

Practical Advice: Listen to your body—it's your most honest guide. Some days, it may crave movement and challenge; other days, it might need rest and gentleness. Embrace both with equal respect. Implementing a "check-in" before each practice can help you assess what you need most at that moment.

Remembering the Joy

Above all, your somatic journey should bring you joy. It's a celebration of connecting with your body and nurturing your well-being.

Practical Advice: Bring elements of play and joy into your practices. Maybe it's practicing yoga poses with a playful spirit, dancing to your favorite songs, or simply enjoying the sensation of the sun on your skin during a mindful walk. Joy can be a powerful motivator and healer.

Your Journey is Uniquely Yours

As you continue on your path, remember that your journey is yours alone—unique, personal, and beautiful in its entirety. The ups and downs, the challenges and triumphs, are all part of the rich tapestry of your experience. Celebrate your resilience, cherish your progress, and keep moving forward with curiosity and compassion. Your commitment to this journey is a testament to your strength and dedication to your well-being. Keep going—you're doing amazing things for yourself, and every step, no matter how small, is a victory.

Adapting Practices for Life Changes

Adapting Somatic Practices to Fit Your Life

Life is a journey of changing stages and circumstances, and your somatic wellness practices can and should evolve with you. Whether you're navigating the busy world of parenthood, moving through the transitions of aging, or adapting to the physical space of a tiny apartment, there's always a way to keep somatic practices a vibrant part of your life. Here's how to adapt and thrive, no matter where you find yourself.

For Busy Parents and Professionals

Finding Time: It can feel impossible to carve out time for somatic practices when you're juggling a million things. But remember, even five minutes counts.

Try This: Incorporate somatic awareness into daily tasks. Practice mindful breathing while doing dishes or waiting for a meeting to start. Turn playtime with the kids into a moment of somatic exploration—notice how your body feels when you're laughing and moving with them.

During Pregnancy and Postpartum

Gentle Adaptations: Your body goes through incredible changes during this time, making it essential to adapt your practices to support what you're experiencing.

Try This: Focus on gentle stretching and breathwork that supports relaxation and connection with your baby. Water-based somatic practices like gentle swimming or water aerobics can be wonderfully supportive and soothing during pregnancy.

Navigating Aging and Mobility Changes

Accessibility: As the body ages, some movements might not feel as accessible as they once were. This doesn't mean somatic practices are off-limits—quite the opposite.

Try This: Chair yoga or tai chi can be excellent for maintaining flexibility and strength without strain. Prioritize practices that enhance balance and joint health.

And always, listen to your body's wisdom, allowing it to guide your activities.

Living in Small Spaces

Space Constraints: Not everyone has the luxury of a dedicated space for somatic practices, but lack of space need not be a barrier.

Try This: Focus on practices that require minimal room, such as seated meditation, breathwork, or standing yoga poses. Use furniture creatively—a chair for balance during yoga, or the edge of a bed for seated stretches.

For Those Experiencing High Stress or Burnout

Stress Reduction: When you're feeling overwhelmed, somatic practices can be a haven, helping to manage stress and restore balance.

Try This: Engage in slow, mindful movements paired with deep breathing to help calm the nervous system. Progressive muscle relaxation can be particularly effective before bed to ease into a restful state.

Adapting to Physical Limitations or Injuries

Personalization: Physical challenges require a thoughtful approach to ensure practices are beneficial and not harmful.

Try This: Work with a specialist, like a physiotherapist or a certified yoga therapist, who can help tailor somatic practices to your needs. Focus on what your body can do, celebrating those movements and sensations, rather than on any limitations.

For Students and Lifelong Learners

Balancing Studies and Wellness: The demands of studies or continuous learning can strain both mind and body, making somatic practices an essential counterbalance.

Try This: Integrate short, mindful breaks between study sessions. A three-minute breathing exercise or a series of neck and shoulder stretches can refresh your mind and relieve physical tension associated with sitting for long periods. Consider walking or cycling to class as part of your somatic practice, using the time to connect with your surroundings and body sensations.

Transitioning Between Careers or Job Loss

Managing Stress and Uncertainty: Career changes or periods of unemployment can be stressful, impacting both emotional and physical well-being.

Try This: Establish a daily routine that includes somatic practices, providing structure and stress relief. Yoga, tai chi, or even mindful walking can help manage anxiety and build resilience. Use somatic practices to cultivate a sense of grounding and stability amidst change, focusing on exercises that promote relaxation and mental clarity.

Entering Retirement

Adjusting to New Rhythms: Retirement marks a significant life transition, with changes in daily routines and possibly increased awareness of aging.

Try This: Explore new somatic activities that fit your interests and physical capabilities, such as joining a dance class, hiking, or gardening. These activities not only keep you physically active but also offer social engagement and a sense of community. Consider practices like Qigong, which can be particularly enriching, offering gentle movements that improve balance, flexibility, and mental well-being.

Dealing with Chronic Illness or Long-term Recovery

Supporting Healing and Comfort: Chronic conditions or long-term recovery from illness or surgery require adjustments to your somatic practice to support healing and manage discomfort.

Try This: Focus on gentle, restorative practices that honor your body's current state, such as guided visualizations that promote healing, gentle yoga or Pilates adapted to your ability, and breathwork to ease pain and anxiety. Collaboration with healthcare providers can ensure your practice supports your health needs.

Living Through Seasonal Changes

Adapting to the Seasons: The changing seasons can affect our energy levels, mood, and physical comfort, inviting adjustments to our somatic practices.

Try This: In warmer months, take advantage of outdoor activities like swimming or early morning walks to connect with nature and revitalize your body. During colder seasons, indoor practices like yoga, Pilates, or dance can keep you active and engaged. Seasonal affective disorder (SAD) can be mitigated through practices that focus on light exposure, such as outdoor walks in natural daylight or exercises near a window.

Keeping Your Practice Alive Through All Seasons of Life

The essence of somatic practices is the deep connection with and listening to your body. As your life changes, let your practices change with you. They can be as dynamic and adaptable as you need them to be.

Remember, the goal is not perfection or performance but presence and awareness. Celebrate your ability to adapt and explore the myriad ways you can maintain this connection to your body and your well-being, no matter the circumstances. Your practice is a reflection of your life: unique, personal, and always evolving. Keep exploring with kindness and curiosity, and know that your somatic journey is yours to shape and enjoy, every step of the way.

Chapter 8: Somatic Wellness for Specific Needs

Somatic exercises for specific conditions

Tailoring somatic exercises to address specific conditions such as chronic pain or stress management involves creating a practice that respects your body's needs while promoting healing and relief. The key is to approach these practices with gentleness, patience, and a focus on what feels beneficial for you. Here's how to adapt somatic exercises to help with chronic pain and stress, always keeping in mind the uniqueness of your experience and needs.

For Chronic Pain

Gentle Movement: Start with gentle, low-impact movements that focus on flexibility and strength without straining your body. Yoga and tai chi are excellent for this, as they combine mindful movements with breathwork, enhancing body awareness and reducing tension.

- **Try This**: In yoga, focus on poses that gently stretch and mobilize the areas of your body where you experience pain, but be careful not to push into discomfort. Tai chi movements are fluid and can be very soothing for the nervous system.

Body Scan Meditation: This practice can help you develop a deeper awareness of your body and the sensations of pain, allowing you to respond to your pain with mindfulness rather than stress.

- **Try This**: Lie down in a comfortable position, close your eyes, and gradually shift your attention through different parts of your body. Notice any sensations without judgment. If you encounter areas of pain, acknowledge them and envision your breath flowing to these areas, gently easing the pain.

Progressive Muscle Relaxation (PMR): PMR can help reduce the tension that often accompanies chronic pain, teaching your body to recognize and release unnecessary muscular tension.

- **Try This**: Tense each muscle group in your body for 5 seconds (without causing pain), then release for 30 seconds, noticing the contrast between tension and relaxation. Start from your toes and move up to your head.

For Stress Management

Mindful Breathing: Deep, mindful breathing activates the parasympathetic nervous system, promoting relaxation and reducing stress levels.

- **Try This**: Practice diaphragmatic breathing, focusing on making your exhales twice as long as your inhales. This can quickly help calm your mind and reduce stress.

Dynamic Movement and Release: Engaging in dynamic movements or exercises can help release the physical manifestations of stress in the body, such as tight muscles and restricted breathing.

- **Try This**: Incorporate movements that open up the chest and shoulders, areas where stress is commonly held. Dancing or any form of expressive movement can also be incredibly liberating and stress-relieving.

Guided Imagery and Visualization: Using your mind to visualize calming and peaceful images can have a profound effect on reducing stress levels, leveraging the mind-body connection.

- **Try This**: Sit or lie in a comfortable position and imagine a peaceful scene—perhaps a quiet beach, a serene forest, or a mountain stream. Engage all your senses in this visualization, and breathe deeply as you immerse yourself in the calmness of your chosen setting.

For Anxiety

Focused Breathing Exercises: Anxiety can make your breath shallow and rapid, heightening feelings of panic. Focused breathing exercises can help regulate your breathing and calm your nervous system.

- **Try This**: Practice the "Box Breathing" technique, where you inhale for a count of four, hold for four, exhale for four, and hold again for four. This pattern can help slow down your breathing and focus your mind, reducing anxiety.

Grounding Techniques: Anxiety can often make you feel untethered or disconnected from the present. Grounding techniques can help bring you back to the here and now.

- **Try This**: Engage in a grounding exercise by noticing five things you can see, four things you can touch, three things you can hear, two things you can smell, and one thing you can taste. This practice helps anchor you in the present moment, easing anxious thoughts.

For Insomnia

Relaxation Before Bed: Preparing your body for sleep with somatic practices can improve the quality of your rest, addressing insomnia at its roots.

- **Try This**: Engage in gentle, restorative yoga or simple stretching before bed to release physical tension. Combine this with deep, diaphragmatic breathing to signal to your body that it's time to wind down.

Mindful Body Scans: A mindful body scan can help calm an overactive mind, making it easier to fall asleep.

- **Try This**: In bed, slowly shift your attention through different parts of your body, from your toes up to your head. Focus on releasing tension in each area as you go, encouraging a state of relaxation conducive to sleep.

For Recovery from Injury

Gentle, Adaptive Movement: When recovering from an injury, it's crucial to keep the body moving in safe, gentle ways to maintain flexibility and prevent stiffness, without putting strain on the injury.

- **Try This**: Work with a physical therapist to identify safe somatic exercises that target areas around the injury, promoting blood flow and healing. Water-based exercises can also be especially beneficial for low-impact movement.

Visualization for Healing: The mind-body connection is powerful, and visualization can play a significant role in your recovery process.

- **Try This**: Visualize the injured area healing and becoming stronger with each breath you take. This not only aids in relaxation but can also positively impact your physical recovery by focusing your body's attention on the healing process.

General Tips for Tailoring Somatic Practices

- **Listen to Your Body**: Always be attuned to what your body is telling you. If something feels wrong or painful, stop and adjust accordingly. Healing and wellness are about nurturing your body, not pushing through pain.

- **Stay Consistent but Flexible**: Consistency in practice can greatly aid in managing chronic conditions, but be flexible in your approach. Some days may require a gentler practice than others, and that's perfectly okay.
- **Seek Professional Guidance**: For chronic conditions or specific challenges, consulting with healthcare professionals can provide you with tailored advice and ensure your practices support your health and recovery.

Adapting Practices for Your Needs

When tailoring somatic exercises for specific conditions, the most important thing is to listen to your body and respect its limits. Each day might be different, and that's okay. Be willing to adjust your practices based on how you're feeling at any given moment.

For chronic conditions, it might also be beneficial to consult with healthcare professionals, such as a physical therapist or a pain specialist, who can provide guidance on which somatic practices may be most beneficial for you.

Remember, somatic exercises are not just about physical movement; they're about cultivating a deeper connection with your body, learning to listen to its signals, and responding with kindness and care. By adapting these practices to your specific needs, you're taking an active role in your own healing and well-being.

Somatic Practices for Emotional Well-being and Recovery

Embracing somatic practices extends beyond physical wellness into the realm of emotional healing and recovery from life's stresses. Whether you're facing grief, burnout, or the challenge of adapting to major life changes, somatic practices can be personalized to support resilience and recovery. Here's how to further tailor these practices to meet the demands of various emotional states and life events.

For Grief and Loss

Mindful Walking in Nature: Grief can make the world feel heavy and dark. Mindful walking in nature allows you to connect with the larger cycle of life and death, offering a broader perspective and a sense of continuity.

- **Try This**: As you walk, pay attention to the life around you—the plants, animals, and changing seasons. Allow yourself to feel part of this natural cycle, finding comfort in the constancy of change.

Breathwork for Release: Grief often resides deeply in the body, manifesting as tightness in the chest or a lump in the throat. Breathwork can help release these physical manifestations of grief.

- **Try This**: Practice deep, controlled breathing exercises, focusing on exhaling fully to release the grief held within. Imagine each exhale carrying away a bit of your pain, making space for healing and new beginnings.

For Burnout

Yoga Nidra for Deep Rest: Burnout drains your energy and dims your spirit. Yoga Nidra, a form of guided relaxation, offers deep rest and rejuvenation, addressing the root of burnout by replenishing your mental and emotional reserves.

- **Try This**: Find a guided Yoga Nidra session (many are available online for free). Allow yourself to be led through this "yogic sleep," reaching a state of consciousness between waking and sleeping that is profoundly restorative.

Creative Movement to Reignite Passion: Burnout can leave you feeling disconnected from your passions and creativity. Engaging in free, expressive movement can help reignite these sparks.

- **Try This**: Put on music that moves you and allow your body to express itself freely through dance. Don't worry about technique or appearance; focus on the joy of movement and the reawakening of your creative spirit.

For Major Life Transitions

Tai Chi for Balance and Centering: Major life changes, whether positive or negative, can throw off your sense of balance. Tai Chi emphasizes slow, deliberate movements that can help restore your internal sense of equilibrium.

- **Try This**: Begin with simple Tai Chi exercises, focusing on the flow of movement and breath. Let this practice be a metaphor for finding balance amid life's changes, moving through them with grace and intention.

Somatic Journaling for Reflection and Clarity: During times of transition, it's helpful to reflect on your experiences and emotions. Somatic journaling combines body awareness with written reflection, offering insights into how your body is processing these changes.

- **Try This**: After a somatic practice, take a few minutes to journal about your experience. How does your body feel? What emotions are present? How are these sensations connected to the changes in your life? This practice can provide clarity and direction during uncertain times.

Embracing Adaptability in Your Somatic Practice

Adapting your somatic practice to your life's current chapter is about honoring where you are right now and meeting yourself with compassion and understanding. Whether you're navigating grief, burnout, or transitions, remember that your practice is a supportive friend, there to hold space for you in every season of life.

Above all, give yourself permission to explore and adjust your practice as needed. What works one day may not feel right the next, and that's perfectly okay. The goal is to maintain a dialogue with your body and emotions, using somatic practices as tools for healing, grounding, and rejuvenation. Your journey is uniquely yours, and your practice can be a reflection of your resilience, adaptability, and growth.

Case studies and testimonials

Case Study: Emily's Journey Through Stress Management with Somatic Practices

Background: Emily, a 38-year-old project manager in a bustling marketing firm, found herself overwhelmed by stress. Long hours, tight deadlines, and constant digital connectivity left her feeling anxious and disconnected from her own body. She noticed a persistent tightness in her shoulders, trouble sleeping, and an inability to relax even in her downtime.

Intervention: After attending a workshop on mindfulness and somatic wellness, Emily decided to integrate somatic practices into her daily routine. She started with two key practices: mindful breathing and gentle yoga, focusing on reconnecting with her body and managing stress.

Mindful Breathing: Emily began her day with a five-minute mindful breathing exercise. Sitting quietly each morning, she focused on her breath, noticing the rise and fall of her chest, the cool air entering her nostrils, and the warmer air exhaling. This practice helped her set a calm, centered tone for the day.

Gentle Yoga: In the evenings, Emily engaged in a 20-minute gentle yoga session. She focused on poses that released tension in her shoulders and back, areas where she held most of her stress. Through yoga, she learned to listen to her body, adapting poses to what felt right each day.

Results: After several weeks, Emily noticed significant changes. Her shoulder tension decreased, her sleep improved, and she felt more present and engaged during her workday. The mindful breathing became a tool she used throughout the day, taking short breaks to center herself when work pressure mounted.

Testimonial: "Incorporating somatic practices into my routine has been transformative," Emily shared. "I've learned to recognize when stress is creeping in and have tools to manage it before it overwhelms me. Yoga has not only eased my physical tension but has taught me patience and acceptance—of my body's limitations and my own. I feel like I've rediscovered a sense of calm and connection I hadn't realized I'd lost."

Case Study: Alex's Recovery from Chronic Pain Through Somatic Awareness

Background: Alex, a 45-year-old graphic designer, had been dealing with chronic lower back pain for years. The pain affected his work, his mood, and his overall quality of life. Traditional treatments provided temporary relief, but the pain always returned, leaving Alex feeling frustrated and hopeless.

Intervention: After researching alternative approaches, Alex decided to explore somatic practices, specifically body scan meditation and somatic movement, to address his chronic pain.

Body Scan Meditation: Each night before bed, Alex practiced body scan meditation, gradually shifting his attention through different parts of his body. This practice helped him develop a heightened awareness of where he held tension and how it contributed to his pain.

Somatic Movement: Alex also incorporated somatic movement into his daily routine. Working with a somatic therapist, he learned movements that specifically targeted his lower back, gently stretching and strengthening the area without exacerbating the pain.

Results: Over time, Alex began to notice a decrease in his pain levels. More importantly, he developed a deeper understanding of his body's signals. He learned to adjust his movements throughout the day to avoid tension build-up, and the body scan meditation provided him with a tool to release stress and tension before it affected his back.

Testimonial: "I never realized how disconnected I was from my own body," Alex reflected. "Through somatic practices, I've not only seen an improvement in my pain but also in my relationship with my body. I feel more in tune with its needs, and for the first time in years, I'm hopeful about managing my pain long-term. It's like I've been given a new lease on life."

Case Study: Liam's Overcoming Insomnia with Somatic Practices

Background: Liam, a 52-year-old school teacher, struggled with insomnia for several years. Night after night, he lay awake, cycling through worry and frustration, which only seemed to make sleep more elusive. His daytime energy was plummeting, affecting his work and personal life.

Intervention: Desperate for a solution, Liam turned to somatic practices after reading about their benefits for sleep disorders. He focused on two main strategies: progressive muscle relaxation (PMR) and guided somatic meditation focused on sleep.

Progressive Muscle Relaxation (PMR): Liam began incorporating PMR into his nightly routine. Lying in bed, he would tense each muscle group for a few seconds, then release, working his way from his toes to his forehead. This helped him become more aware of physical tension and how to consciously relax his muscles.

Guided Somatic Meditation: Additionally, Liam listened to guided somatic meditations designed to prepare the mind and body for sleep. These meditations included visualizations of peaceful, restful places and instructions to bring awareness to and then relax different parts of the body.

Results: Within a few weeks, Liam noticed a significant improvement in his ability to fall asleep and stay asleep. The practices helped him break the cycle of anxiety about sleep, allowing him to approach bedtime with a sense of calm instead of dread.

Testimonial: "I had almost given up hope of ever getting a good night's sleep again," Liam admitted. "Learning to tune into my body and relax it on purpose was a game-changer. I'm not just sleeping better; I feel like I've regained control over my life. It's amazing how something as simple as being more in touch with my body could have such a profound impact."

Case Study: Sophia's Journey from Burnout to Balance with Somatic Yoga

Background: Sophia, a 30-year-old software developer, was on the brink of burnout. The relentless pace of her job, combined with the isolation of working remotely, left her feeling drained and disconnected from her sense of self.

Intervention: Seeking a holistic way to manage her stress and reconnect with her body, Sophia began practicing somatic yoga, a form of yoga that emphasizes internal perception and the experience of movement.

Somatic Yoga: Sophia attended a weekly somatic yoga class, where the focus was on noticing the sensations within her body during each pose and movement, rather than achieving perfect form. This practice encouraged her to pay attention to her body's needs and limits, promoting a sense of mindfulness and presence she found lacking in her daily life.

Integration into Daily Routine: Beyond the weekly classes, Sophia integrated short somatic yoga sequences into her morning routine, setting a grounded, centered tone for her day. She also practiced somatic breathing exercises during work breaks, using them as moments of reconnection and relaxation amidst the chaos of her job.

Results: Over several months, Sophia experienced a profound shift in her mental and emotional well-being. Her stress levels decreased noticeably, and she found herself approaching her work with more calmness and clarity. The practices also rekindled her passion for her job, helping her find a healthier work-life balance.

Testimonial: "Somatic yoga didn't just help me manage stress; it transformed the way I relate to my body and my work," Sophia shared. "I've learned to listen to my body's signals, taking breaks when I need them and approaching my tasks with a sense of presence and mindfulness. It feels like I've found my way back to myself."

Concluding Thoughts

These narratives underscore the transformative potential of somatic practices in addressing common yet deeply impactful issues like stress and chronic pain. Emily's and Alex's stories highlight the importance of body awareness, the power of mindfulness, and the value of personalizing one's approach to wellness. Through somatic practices, both found not just relief from their symptoms but also a deeper connection to their bodies and a more empowered approach to their well-being.

In addition,the stories of Liam and Sophia illustrate the transformative power of somatic practices in addressing not only physical discomforts, such as insomnia, but also the mental and emotional challenges of burnout. By fostering a deeper connection with their bodies, both found pathways to healing that transcended traditional remedies, highlighting the integral role of somatic awareness in overall well-being. These narratives serve as compelling testimony to the effectiveness of somatic practices in navigating life's challenges, offering hope and practical strategies to those seeking holistic paths to wellness.

Part IV: Sustaining Your Transformation

Chapter 9: Building a Supportive Environment

Creating a Wellness-Supportive Environment

Creating a physical and social environment that nurtures somatic wellness involves thoughtful choices about your surroundings and the people you interact with. Here's some advice on crafting spaces and building relationships that foster a deep connection with your body and mind.

Cultivating Your Physical Space

1. Simplify Your Surroundings: Clutter can be a significant source of stress and distraction. By simplifying your environment, you create a peaceful space where you can focus on your somatic practices without external chaos.

- **Action Step**: Start by decluttering the area where you plan to practice. This doesn't mean your space needs to be sparse or minimalist—just organized in a way that feels calming to you.

2. Bring Nature Inside: Incorporating elements of nature into your space can have a soothing effect, making it easier to connect with your body and the present moment.

- **Action Step**: Consider adding indoor plants, natural light, or even nature sounds to your practice area. These elements can enhance your sense of well-being and deepen your somatic experience.

3. Personalize Your Practice Area: Personal touches can make your practice space feel safe and inviting, encouraging regular engagement with your somatic exercises.

- **Action Step**: Decorate your space with items that inspire you or bring you joy—photos, inspirational quotes, or anything that resonates with your personal journey.

Nurturing Supportive Relationships

1. Communicate Your Needs: Sharing your wellness goals and needs with friends and family can help them understand and support your somatic journey.

- **Action Step**: Have open conversations about the importance of your practice and how loved ones can support you, whether that's respecting your practice time or joining you in mindfulness activities.

2. Seek Like-minded Communities: Connecting with others who share your interest in somatic wellness can provide motivation, inspiration, and a sense of belonging.

- **Action Step**: Look for local groups or online communities that focus on somatic practices like yoga, tai chi, or meditation. Attend workshops or events to deepen your practice and meet peers.

3. Set Boundaries for Wellness: Protecting your time and energy is crucial for maintaining a somatic practice, especially in today's fast-paced world.

- **Action Step**: Learn to say no to commitments that don't align with your wellness goals or that might drain your energy. Setting these boundaries allows you to prioritize your somatic practice and overall well-being.

Integrating Wellness into Your Daily Routine

1. Make Somatic Practices Accessible: Keeping your practice simple and accessible will help you integrate it into your daily life, even on busy days.

- **Action Step**: Prepare a small, go-to set of practices that you can do anywhere, anytime. This might include breathing exercises, a short series of stretches, or mindfulness techniques.

2. Create Wellness Rituals: Building rituals around your somatic practices can help turn them into a cherished part of your routine.

- **Action Step**: Establish rituals that signal the beginning and end of your practice, such as lighting a candle, brewing a cup of herbal tea, or journaling about your experience.

3. Embrace Flexibility: Being flexible with your somatic practice helps you stay committed without feeling pressured or stressed.

- **Action Step**: Allow yourself the freedom to adapt your practice as needed. Some days, you might dive deep into a full routine, while on others, a few mindful breaths might be all you can manage—and that's perfectly okay.

Creating a supportive environment for somatic wellness is about making intentional choices that align with your personal needs and values. By crafting a serene physical space, nurturing positive relationships, and integrating wellness into your daily life, you can build a foundation that supports and enriches your somatic journey. Remember, the goal is to enhance your connection with yourself and your environment in a way that feels authentic and sustainable for you.

Community and relationships in wellness

The role of community and relationships in sustaining wellness cannot be overstated. Human beings are inherently social creatures, and the connections we forge with others play a crucial part in our overall health and well-being. In the context of somatic wellness, community and relationships offer support, inspiration, and a sense of belonging that can significantly enhance our journey. Let's dive into how these elements contribute to sustaining wellness and how you can actively cultivate them in your life.

The Supportive Power of Community

Shared Experience: Engaging with a community of like-minded individuals provides a shared space for experiences and growth. Whether it's a yoga class, a meditation group, or an online forum dedicated to somatic practices, being part of a community offers validation and understanding that you're not alone in your journey.

- **Action Step**: Seek out local or virtual groups that align with your somatic interests. Attend workshops or community events to deepen your connection and learn from the collective wisdom.

Motivation and Accountability: It's easier to stay committed to your wellness practices when you're part of a group with similar goals. The encouragement from community members can boost your motivation, and the accountability can help maintain consistency in your practice.

- **Action Step**: Partner with a friend or group member to share goals and progress. This could be as simple as a weekly check-in to discuss challenges, celebrate successes, and encourage each other to keep going.

The Nurturing Influence of Relationships

Emotional Support: Strong relationships provide emotional support, which is essential during challenging times. Having someone to turn to, who listens and understands, can make a significant difference in managing stress and maintaining mental and emotional health.

- **Action Step**: Cultivate relationships where emotional support is mutual. Be open about your needs and be there for others, creating a supportive exchange that enriches both your wellness journey and theirs.

Inspiration and Growth: Relationships can be a source of inspiration and personal growth. Seeing the progress and resilience of those around you can inspire you to explore new aspects of your own wellness journey and challenge yourself in healthy ways.

- **Action Step**: Engage in conversations about wellness and personal growth with friends and family. Share resources, insights, and experiences that have been meaningful to you.

Cultivating a Wellness-oriented Community

Create Your Own Space: If you can't find an existing community that resonates with you, consider creating your own. This could be an informal gathering of friends interested in wellness or a more structured group that meets regularly for somatic practices.

- **Action Step**: Use social media or community bulletin boards to invite others to join you in a wellness journey. Set a regular time and place for meetings, whether in-person or virtual, and plan activities that align with your collective goals.

Volunteer or Participate in Wellness Events: Volunteering for wellness-related events or participating in community wellness days can broaden your network and deepen your sense of belonging to a wellness-oriented community.

- **Action Step**: Look for opportunities to volunteer at local health fairs, wellness retreats, or workshops. Not only will you contribute to your community, but you'll also connect with others who share your values.

Embracing the Role of Community and Relationships

The journey to somatic wellness is deeply personal, yet it's enriched immeasurably by the presence of a supportive community and nurturing relationships. These connections offer a mirror to our own experiences, providing insights, encouragement, and a reminder of the universal desire for health and happiness. By actively seeking out and contributing to a community, you not only enhance your own wellness journey but also become a beacon of support and inspiration for others on their path.

Chapter 10: Continuing Your Journey

Congratulations on reaching this point in your somatic wellness journey. By now, you've laid a strong foundation and experienced the transformative power of connecting deeply with your body. However, the journey doesn't end here. It's a lifelong path of exploration, learning, and growth. In this chapter, we'll explore resources for further exploration and offer encouragement to keep adapting and deepening your somatic practices.

Resources for Further Exploration

Books:

1. **"The Body Keeps the Score" by Bessel van der Kolk** - A groundbreaking exploration of how trauma affects the body and mind, and how somatic practices can aid in recovery.

2. **"Waking the Tiger" by Peter A. Levine** - Offers insight into healing trauma through somatic experiencing, a practice focusing on bodily sensations.

3. **"Coming to Our Senses" by Jon Kabat-Zinn** - A comprehensive guide on mindfulness and its role in healing and well-being, from the pioneer of Mindfulness-Based Stress Reduction (MBSR).

4. **"Move Your DNA" by Katy Bowman** - Highlights the importance of movement in our daily lives and

offers practical advice for incorporating more natural movement.

Courses:

1. **Mindfulness-Based Stress Reduction (MBSR)** - Check for local or online MBSR courses, a structured program that integrates mindfulness meditation and somatic practices.

2. **Yoga Teacher Training** - Even if you don't plan to teach, a yoga teacher training course can deepen your understanding of the somatic aspects of yoga.

3. **Tai Chi or Qigong Classes** - Many community centers or wellness studios offer classes in these gentle martial arts, known for their health benefits and focus on body awareness.

Communities:

1. **Meetup Groups**: Websites like Meetup.com can connect you with local groups practicing yoga, meditation, tai chi, and other somatic disciplines.

2. **Online Forums and Social Media**: Platforms like Reddit or specific Facebook groups can be valuable resources for sharing experiences, asking questions, and finding support.

3. **Retreats and Workshops**: Attending a retreat or workshop can be a powerful way to deepen your

practice and connect with a community of like-minded individuals.

Keep Exploring and Adapting

Your somatic journey is uniquely yours, shaped by your experiences, challenges, and discoveries. As you move forward, remember to:

- **Stay Curious**: Always be open to learning and trying new practices. What resonates with you today might evolve tomorrow. Embrace the journey of discovery with an open heart and mind.

- **Listen to Your Body**: Your body is your most honest guide. Continue to cultivate a deep listening to its signals and needs, adjusting your practices accordingly.

- **Be Patient and Compassionate**: Some days will feel like a step forward, others a step back. Treat yourself with kindness and patience, recognizing that growth often happens in the most unexpected ways.

- **Share Your Journey**: Sharing your experiences can not only enrich your own journey but also inspire and support others on theirs. Whether it's through social media, blogging, or simply talking with friends, don't underestimate the value of your insight.

Final Thoughts

As you continue your journey, remember that somatic wellness is not a destination but a way of living. It's about continuously deepening your connection with your body, learning from its wisdom, and allowing that knowledge to guide you toward greater health and happiness. The resources and communities available to you are as vast as they are varied, offering endless opportunities for growth and connection. Keep exploring, keep learning, and most importantly, keep feeling. Your journey is an endless horizon of possibility—embrace it with open arms and an open heart.

Conclusion

Reflecting on Your Journey

As you stand at this pivotal moment, looking back over the last 30 days, it's time to reflect on the transformation you've undergone through your dedication to somatic wellness. This journey has likely been one of discovery, challenge, and growth, offering you insights not just into your physical being but into your emotional and mental landscapes as well. Let's summarize the transformation you've experienced and envision the path that lies ahead.

The Transformation

Increased Body Awareness: One of the most profound changes you may have noticed is a deeper connection with your body. Perhaps you're more attuned to its signals now, whether it's recognizing the early signs of stress or identifying what brings you physical joy and comfort.

Emotional Resilience: Through somatic practices, you've likely developed tools for navigating your emotions more effectively. This might manifest as a newfound calmness in the face of stress or a deeper understanding and acceptance of your emotional responses.

Improved Physical Well-being: Whether your goal was to manage pain, enhance flexibility, or simply feel more grounded, you've likely seen changes in your physical well-being. These changes might include reduced tension, greater mobility, or an overall sense of physical vitality.

Mindfulness and Presence: The somatic journey encourages a mindful approach to life, teaching you to live more fully in the present moment. This might have transformed how you experience daily life, from how you eat and work to how you communicate with others.

Looking Ahead

As you move forward from these initial 30 days, consider how you can continue to integrate and deepen these practices in your life.

Setting New Goals: With the foundation you've built, now is the time to set new goals for your continued somatic journey. Perhaps there's a specific practice you want to explore further or a new aspect of wellness you're curious about.

Incorporating Variety: To keep your practice vibrant and engaging, consider incorporating new somatic exercises or exploring different aspects of wellness. This might mean trying a new type of movement, like dance or martial arts, or deepening your meditation practice.

Continuing Education: The field of somatic wellness is vast and rich with knowledge. Continue your education through books, courses, and workshops to keep growing and evolving in your practice.

Building Community: Remember, the journey is enriched by sharing it with others. Continue to seek out and contribute to communities that resonate with your path, whether online or in person.

Sustaining Your Transformation

Embrace Lifelong Learning: Your body is an incredible teacher, and there is always more to learn from it. Stay curious about what it can teach you. This might mean delving deeper into the science of somatic practices, exploring new techniques, or even training to guide others on their somatic journeys.

- **Action Step**: Consider enrolling in advanced workshops or certification programs related to somatic practices. This could enhance your own practice and potentially open new pathways for sharing these transformative experiences with others.

Cultivate Daily Practices: Integrating somatic practices into your daily routine ensures that your journey continues to evolve. This doesn't mean setting aside large blocks of time each day; even small, consistent practices can yield profound benefits.

- **Action Step**: Identify two to three somatic exercises that you can easily incorporate into your daily life, such as mindful breathing during your commute or gentle stretching before bed. Make these practices non-negotiable parts of your day.

Deepening Your Transformation

Explore the Interconnection of Mind, Body, and Spirit: As you advance in your somatic journey, you'll discover the deep interconnection between your physical sensations, emotional states, and spiritual well-being. Exploring these connections can lead to profound insights and further personal growth.

- **Action Step**: Dedicate time each week to practices that specifically address the mind-body-spirit connection. This could be through meditation, journaling about your somatic experiences, or engaging in activities that nourish your spirit, like spending time in nature or practicing acts of kindness.

Personalize Your Practice: As you become more attuned to your body's needs and responses, you'll be in a better position to personalize your somatic practices. This personalization is key to maintaining engagement and ensuring that your practice continues to meet your evolving needs.

- **Action Step**: Regularly assess how your current practices are serving you. Don't hesitate to modify them or try new approaches based on what you're learning about yourself. This might mean adjusting the intensity, duration, or even the type of practices you're doing.

Beyond the Individual Journey

Building a Supportive Community: Sharing your journey with others not only enriches your own experience but can also provide support and inspiration to those around you. A community can offer diverse perspectives and collective wisdom, enhancing the depth and breadth of your somatic exploration.

- **Action Step**: If you haven't already, seek out or create a community of practice. This could be a formal group that meets regularly or an informal gathering of friends interested in somatic wellness. Share your experiences, challenges, and insights, and be open to learning from others.

Giving Back: As you grow in your somatic journey, consider ways you can give back to the community that supports you. This might involve volunteering, mentoring, or even sharing your story to inspire others.

- **Action Step**: Look for opportunities to contribute to your community, whether by leading a workshop, offering free classes, or simply being there for someone who is just beginning their somatic journey.

Reflecting on the Path Ahead

The journey of somatic wellness is infinite, filled with continual learning, growth, and transformation. Remember, every moment of awareness, every breath, and every movement is a step on this path. Celebrate how far you've come, and approach the future with a sense of wonder and openness. Your journey is uniquely yours, a beautiful, ever-unfolding exploration of the depth and richness of human experience. Continue to move forward with kindness, curiosity, and a commitment to your well-being.

Final Words of Encouragement

Your journey over the last 30 days is just the beginning. Each day offers a new opportunity to deepen your connection with yourself, to learn, and to grow. Celebrate the progress you've made and approach the future with openness and curiosity. The path of somatic wellness is not linear but a spiral, leading you deeper into the understanding of your body, mind, and spirit. Embrace this journey with kindness towards yourself, knowing that each step, each breath, and each moment of awareness is a testament to your commitment to living a more connected, vibrant life.

Appendices

Templates for tracking progress

Daily Somatic Practice Log

Field	Details
Date	
Time of Practice	
Duration	
Somatic Practices Performed	(e.g., yoga, mindful walking, body scan meditation)
Physical Sensations Noted	(e.g., tension, relaxation, energy levels)
Emotional State Before Practice	
Emotional State After Practice	
Insights Gained	
Adjustments for Tomorrow	

Weekly Reflection Template

Field	Details
Week Ending (Date)	
Overall Emotional Tone	
Physical Well-being Check-in	(any changes in pain, tension, energy levels?)

Most Impactful Practice	
Challenges Faced	
How I Overcame Challenges	
Insights or Patterns Observed	
Goals for Next Week	
Self-Care Actions Taken	

Monthly Overview and Reflection

Field	Details
Month	
Key Achievements	(Include milestones in practice consistency, depth of emotional awareness, physical improvements, etc.)
Most Frequently Used Practices	
New Practices Tried	
Physical and Emotional Changes Noticed	
Challenges Encountered	
How Challenges Were Addressed	

Insights Gained About Self	
Intentions for Next Month	
Additional Notes/Reflections	

Mindfulness and Emotional Well-being Log

Field	**Details**
Date	
Mindfulness Practice	(e.g., seated meditation, mindful eating)
Duration	
Emotional State Before	
Emotional State After	
Specific Thoughts/Feelings Noted	
Areas of Resistance or Ease	
Insights/Reflections	

Physical Activity and Energy Levels Log

Field	Details
Date	
Type of Physical Activity	(e.g., yoga, tai chi, walking)
Duration	
Energy Level Before	(Low, Medium, High)
Energy Level After	(Low, Medium, High)
Physical Sensations Noted	
Overall Mood	
Adjustments for Next Session	

Sleep Quality and Somatic Practices Log

Field	**Details**
Date	
Pre-Sleep Somatic Practice	(e.g., body scan, progressive muscle relaxation)
Duration of Practice	
Sleep Onset Time	
Number of Awakenings	
Wake Up Time	
Sleep Quality (1-10)	
Morning Physical Sensations	
Morning Emotional State	
Reflections/Insights	

Nutrition and Body Awareness Log

Field	Details
Date	
Meals Consumed	(Brief description and time)
Mindful Eating Practice	(Yes/No + details)
Physical Sensations Post-Meal	(e.g., fullness, energy levels)
Emotional State Post-Meal	
Cravings Noted	
Hydration Level	(Number of glasses of water)
Insights/Adjustments Needed	

How to Use These Templates

- **Tailor to Your Needs**: Feel free to customize these templates further based on your personal goals and areas of focus. Adding or removing fields to suit your tracking preferences can make them more relevant and useful for you.

- **Consistency is Key**: Try to fill out the logs regularly to get the most benefit. Consistent tracking can reveal patterns and insights that sporadic logging might miss.

- **Reflect and Adjust**: Use the insights gained from these logs to adjust your practices, lifestyle choices, and routines. This reflective process is where the real growth and understanding occur.

By expanding your tracking to include these various aspects of somatic wellness, you're creating a comprehensive view of your journey. This holistic approach not only enriches your practice but also fosters a deeper connection between your mind, body, and environment, paving the way for sustained well-being and personal growth.

Made in the USA
Monee, IL
04 November 2026

67387465R10075